Understanding the
Mental Health
Problems of
Children and
Adolescents

Related books of interest

Child and Family Practice: A Relational Perspective
Shelley Cohen Konrad

Character Formation and Identity in Adolescence
Randolph L. Lucente

Children and Loss: A Practical Handbook for Professionals
Elizabeth C. Pomeroy and Renée Bradford Garcia

Understanding and Managing the Therapeutic Relationship
Fred R. McKenzie

Interviewing for the Helping Professions: A Relational Approach
Fred McKenzie

Psychoeducation in Mental Health
Joseph Walsh

Evidence-Based Practices for Social Workers: An Interdisciplinary Approach, Second Edition
Thomas O'Hare

Understanding the

Mental Health Problems of Children and Adolescents

Kirstin Painter

MHMR Tarrant

Maria Scannapieco

University of Texas at Arlington

LYCEUM

BOOKS, INC.

Chicago, IL 60637

© 2015 by Lyceum Books, Inc.

Published by
LYCEUM BOOKS, INC.
5758 S. Blackstone Avenue
Chicago, Illinois 60637
773-643-1903 fax
773-643-1902 phone
lyceum@lyceumbooks.com
www.lyceumbooks.com

6   5   4   3   2   1   15   16   17   18   19

ISBN 978-1-933478-88-3

Printed in the United States of America.

Library of Congress Cataloging-in-Publication Data

Painter, Kirstin, 1963- , author.
    Understanding the mental health problems of children and adolescents / Kirstin Painter, Maria Scannapieco.
        p. ; cm.
    Includes bibliographical references.
    ISBN 978-1-933478-88-3 (pbk.)
    I. Scannapieco, Maria, author.   II. Title.
[DNLM: 1. Mental Disorders.   2. Adolescent.   3. Child. WS 350]
RJ503
616.8900835—dc23
                                                                    2014045017

Contents

List of Tables

Foreword

Stumbling through the dense forest, the roots of giant trees
continually tripped me. One day I tripped on yet another root,
but this time I looked up to find the right tree.

THIS IS WHAT IT FEELS LIKE to have a child with mental health problems. If your child has asthma, diabetes, or another illness, you can ask around and find resources, physicians, and treatments. But, even in the second decade of the twenty-first century, mental illnesses remain in dark shadows—seldom mentioned in polite society. Yet, at any given time, one in five children is experiencing some form of mental illness. Mental illnesses must come out of the shadows, but they have a long way to go.

Imagine, if you will, what it must be like to have a child who is violent, using street drugs, sexually active, or out of control. Because the symptoms of mental illnesses are typically behavioral, parents tend to blame themselves for not teaching their children well. And others blame the parents as well. How often have you heard remarks such as, "If her parents just spent more time with her . . . ," "If his parents didn't let him get away with everything . . . ," or "If her parents were more involved, they would know where she is and who she is with"?

As a parent of a child who was diagnosed with bipolar disorder as an adolescent, I can tell you these remarks sting. Perhaps even more stinging, though, is the realization that you might have once said the same things about children and adolescents who seemed out of control: "What is wrong with the parents? Can't they control that child?"

In the next pages, the authors, Kirstin Painter and Maria Scannapieco, will present an excellent discussion on mental illnesses in children and adolescents. They have kindly asked me to write a foreword to give you the perspective of a parent's experiences when a child or adolescent has a mental illness—and ways that you can help.

The first thing a social worker should do is avoid guilt-inducing statements, gestures, or eye rolling when determining the background of a child. Yes, the parents may have been responsible in part for triggering the child's symptoms. However, what good does it do to add guilt on top of guilt? If parents are seeking help for their children, they can't be all bad, can they? Instead, the therapist can help the parents discover their strengths and make a better future for themselves and their children.

Second, social workers need to recognize that parents go through all the stages of grief when learning that their child has a mental illness. What would your reaction be if the child you held in your arms as an infant—the child whose future you dreamed of—were diagnosed with a lifelong illness that could prevent those dreams from coming true? In the earliest stages, parents are often in denial—no matter how educated or accepting they are of mental illnesses. They do not want this for their children. Social workers can play a role in helping parents recognize and navigate through their grief as they work to help their children recover.

It is also common for social workers to become frustrated with parents who will not ensure that their children take prescribed medication. Again, though, put yourself in their place. They have read about children committing suicide after starting antidepressants. The news is big and bold on the front page. Unfortunately, explanations and medical discussions of these issues are buried—if they are included in the news at all. So parents do not always have a wealth of resource information. And they do not turn to their friends because no one ever talks about mental illness—so they feel they must be the only ones grappling with this problem.

It is always important to listen to the parents just as intently as you do to the child or adolescent. The children with mental illnesses whom I have encountered are often among the brightest I have ever known. As such, they know what to say to make themselves look good and their parents look bad. A therapist in a residential treatment center was shocked when my daughter had a full meltdown during family therapy two months into her treatment. Her comment was an incredulous, "I've never seen this child before." My response was, "This is the child I live with every day." Although there were certain satisfactions in having the therapist see what I had been saying, there were still the wasted two months when the behaviors were not addressed because my daughter had never displayed them—despite my having discussed them.

Another role the social worker can play is mediator/facilitator. Too many therapists see the parent/child relationship as antagonistic. It may appear this way because many parents have no way to understand what has been happening. They have been struggling with discipline and may be at their wits' end. There are even some parents who communicate their frustrations to their children, using statements such as, "I've had enough. I give up." The situation may seem antagonistic, and sometimes it is. Often, though, the parents have no idea how to work with an emotionally disturbed child. They blame themselves, but they keep struggling. And all too often social workers present an air of mystery and intrigue: "Thank you for bringing your child to me. Now you just sit out there in the waiting room while we talk." The parent is left totally in the dark, unaware of what is being discussed or—more importantly—what he or she can do to help. The social worker can bring the parent into the room with the child in the last few minutes of the session. This may be a good time to encourage the child to communicate feelings and to discuss the illness openly with the parent and child together. The more parents can be on the same page with the therapist and the child, the more effective the changes at home can be. After all, parents who have been raised in a certain way can find it difficult to suddenly change their parenting styles. But if they understand the benefit to their child, they may feel more empowered to make the changes.

Another aspect of the family to assess and counsel is the situation of other children in the home. Mental illnesses do not affect only the child with the illness—or even the child and parents. Often, a child with mental illness will act out against other children in the family. Parents can be so involved in the care of the child with mental illness that they cannot find the time they need for the other children, which can add to their feelings of guilt. Sometimes a professional can help explain the illness to other children in the family who are old enough to understand. If the family can become more cohesive, it can provide a much better environment for the child struggling with the illness.

Many social workers have advised me to research parenting tools that can work. It's a good idea to arm parents with whatever you can, but never anticipate that typical parenting programs will work. And when they don't, the parents will again feel guilty. They must not have done it correctly or are not capable as parents even when they follow guidelines. For example, many parents try working with privileges. If a child lives up to certain behavioral standards, he or she receives privileges. If not, privileges are removed. In my own case, my daughter would miss the privileges for a very short time and then forget about them. They just didn't matter to her. How do you decide which privileges to remove when the privileges valued by the child change rapidly? The behavior contract is another example of a tool that does not work for every parent. The adolescents you see are often very savvy. They know they just need to sign the contract to move forward, so they do. However, they may have no intention of living up to their promises. Again, the parents feel guilty because they were unable to make the child commit to the terms of the contract.

As you will see in the following pages, knowledge about mental illnesses is constantly changing. When my adopted daughter was just six weeks old—before she came to us—she was physically abused. We knew a little about the abuse when we adopted her, but my thinking was that she would never remember anything that happened at such an early age. Over the years, research has shown that even early childhood trauma can change the way a child's brain develops. That might seem like common sense to you, but parents continue to be unaware of the nature and impact of early childhood trauma. As a social worker, you can help parents understand the importance of those early childhood experiences. I will always wonder if my daughter's behaviors would have become so out of control if we had addressed the trauma issues.

Finally, social workers often try to help parents deal with their child's situation by encouraging the parents to take care of themselves. This is good advice without a doubt. However, parents are often emotionally and financially strapped. Many cannot even afford a movie night out. Single parents may have lost the friends they once had—the parents of their children's friends have busy lives with their healthy children, and sometimes they see the parent of a child with mental illness as flawed. So continue to tell parents to take care of themselves for the sake of their children, but give them some ideas about ways they can do that within the limitations they have.

Although I have addressed many issues in this foreword, I must stress that most of my experiences with social workers have been positive. I consider many of those who worked with my daughter to be life savers. The ones who cared about my entire family and made that clear have my undying gratitude. I have been fortunate to work with many social workers beyond those who provided therapy for my child, including the authors. I have seen firsthand the help they give to families who struggle every day with a child's mental illness. I thank all of them and encourage you to follow their examples and truly make a difference in the lives of children with mental illness and their families.

Kay Barkin
Parent of a child with bipolar disorder
Social marketer for Mental Health Mental Retardation of Tarrant County
Hand in Hand System of Care

Preface

THE OBJECTIVE OF *Understanding the Mental Health Problems of Children and Adolescents* is to provide a practical guide for social workers on promoting positive mental health in youth from a system of care perspective. Social workers will gain an understanding of the scope of mental health issues in youth to include definitions, etiology, and evidence-based treatments, as well as the importance of partnering with youth and caregivers, addressing issues from a strengths perspective, and engaging in culturally sensitive practice.

Social workers in all fields of practice need this information. This book is distinctive in its clear presentation and explanation of the various mental health problems and the treatment for these problems. We begin our book with a foreword from a parent of a child who has experienced mental health problems. We think this is important because we need the voices of our parents and youth to fully understand their experiences. The book also includes the core competencies of the Council on Social Work Education and a table outlining the competencies that are addressed in each chapter.

The first three chapters set the context of the book. We discuss the state of mental illness in the United States and the changes to the *Diagnostic and Statistical Manual of Mental Disorders* from version IV-TR to version 5. The theoretical framework of the book is outlined for understanding and treating mental health problems. A brief overview of child and adolescent development is provided as a refresher for the reader.

The remaining chapters are divided by disorder and treatment. For each mental health problem area, there is a chapter dedicated to the definition and etiology of the disorder followed by a second chapter that describes the known treatments for the disorder. Case scenarios are presented with discussion questions to help guide application of the chapter content. Comorbidity with substance abuse is also discussed. Because secondary educational settings are key to identifying and treating mental health problems for youth and adolescents, the final chapter focuses on educational programs and practices.

Evidence-based and informed practice is emphasized throughout the book. There is a great disparity between the evidence base of effective community-based treatments for youth with mental health disorders and the treatments available to these youth. Although the concept of evidence-based practice has gained increased attention over the past twenty years, the profession of social work began incorporating evidence-based practice models into the professional literature in 2003. Today, the literature is increasingly emphasizing the importance of evidence-based practices. Unfortunately, although there has been an increase in the literature emphasizing the importance of evidence-based programs and treatments and early identification and treatment of youth with mental health problems, social work lacks adequate training in mental health issues of children and evidence-based practices.

To enhance the learning experience, have your students access the National Institute of Mental Health website to view illustrations of the brain and how it functions (nimh.nih.gov/news/image-library). This is particularly applicable in chapters 3, 4, and 14. You will find illustrations of normal brain development as well as comparisons to brains experiencing mental illness and trauma.

The appendix provides website links to various resources that will support continued learning in mental health. It is the authors' hope that the materials in the book are straightforward and immediately applicable to practice.

Council on Social Work Education Educational Policy and Accreditation Standards: Core Competencies

THE COUNCIL OF SOCIAL WORK adopted in 2008 and revised in 2010 the Educational Policy and Accreditation Standards. These standards lay out ten core social work competencies guiding curriculum design in social work education programs. Competencies are practice behaviors integrating knowledge, values, and skills.

The competencies covered in this book are outlined below, followed by a matrix that shows the competencies that are covered in each chapter.

EDUCATIONAL POLICY 2.1.1

Identify as a professional social worker and conduct oneself accordingly.

Social workers serve as representatives of the profession, its mission, and its core values. They know the profession's history. Social workers commit themselves to the profession's enhancement and to their own professional conduct and growth. Social workers

- Advocate for client access to the services of social work;
- Practice personal reflection and self-correction to assure continual professional development;
- Attend to professional roles and boundaries;
- Demonstrate professional demeanor in behavior, appearance, and communication;

- Engage in career-long learning;
- Use supervision and consultation.

EDUCATIONAL POLICY 2.1.2

Apply social work ethical principles to guide professional practice.

Social workers have an obligation to conduct themselves ethically and to engage in ethical decision-making. Social workers are knowledgeable about the value base of the profession, its ethical standards, and relevant law. Social workers

- Recognize and manage personal values in a way that allows professional values to guide practice;
- Make ethical decisions by applying standards of the National Association of Social Workers Code of Ethics and, as applicable, of the International Federation of Social Workers/International Association of Schools of Social Work Ethics in Social Work, Statement of Principles;
- Tolerate ambiguity in resolving ethical conflicts;
- Apply strategies of ethical reasoning to arrive at principled decisions.

EDUCATIONAL POLICY 2.1.3

Apply critical thinking to inform and communicate professional judgments.

Social workers are knowledgeable about the principles of logic, scientific inquiry, and reasoned discernment. They use critical thinking augmented by creativity and curiosity. Critical thinking also requires the synthesis and communication of relevant information. Social workers

- Distinguish, appraise, and integrate multiple sources of knowledge, including research-based knowledge, and practice wisdom;
- Analyze models of assessment, prevention, intervention, and evaluation;
- Demonstrate effective oral and written communication in working with individuals, families, groups, organizations, communities, and colleagues.

EDUCATIONAL POLICY 2.1.4

Engage diversity and difference in practice.

Social workers understand how diversity characterizes and shapes the human experience and is critical to the formation of identity. The dimensions of diversity are understood as the intersectionality of multiple factors including age, class, color, culture, disability, ethnicity, gender, gender identity and expression, immigration status, political ideology, race, religion, sex, and sexual orientation. Social workers appreciate that, as a consequence of difference, a person's life experiences may include oppression, poverty, marginalization, and alienation as well as privilege, power, and acclaim. Social workers

- Recognize the extent to which a culture's structures and values may oppress, marginalize, alienate, or create or enhance privilege and power;
- Gain sufficient self-awareness to eliminate the influence of personal biases and values in working with diverse groups;
- Recognize and communicate their understanding of the importance of difference in shaping life experiences;
- View themselves as learners and engage those with whom they work as informants.

EDUCATIONAL POLICY 2.1.5

Advance human rights and social and economic justice.

Each person, regardless of position in society, has basic human rights, such as freedom, safety, privacy, an adequate standard of living, health care, and education. Social workers recognize the global interconnections of oppression and are knowledgeable about theories of justice and strategies to promote human and civil rights. Social work incorporates social justice practices in organizations, institutions, and society to ensure that these basic human rights are distributed equitably and without prejudice. Social workers

- Understand the forms and mechanisms of oppression and discrimination;
- Advocate for human rights and social and economic justice;
- Engage in practices that advance social and economic justice.

EDUCATIONAL POLICY 2.1.6

Engage in research-informed practice and practice-informed research.

Social workers use practice experience to inform research; employ evidence-based interventions; evaluate their own practice; and use research findings to improve practice, policy, and social service delivery. Social workers comprehend quantitative and qualitative research and understand scientific and ethical approaches to building knowledge. Social workers

- Use practice experience to inform scientific inquiry;
- Use research evidence to inform practice.

EDUCATIONAL POLICY 2.1.7

Apply knowledge of human behavior and the social environment.

Social workers are knowledgeable about human behavior across the life course, the range of social systems in which people live, and the ways social systems promote or deter people in maintaining or achieving health and well-being. Social workers apply theories and knowledge from the liberal arts to understand biological, social, cultural, psychological, and spiritual development. Social workers

- Utilize conceptual frameworks to guide the processes of assessment, intervention, and evaluation;
- Critique and apply knowledge to understand person and environment.

EDUCATIONAL POLICY 2.1.8

Engage in policy practice to advance social and economic well-being and to deliver effective social work services.

Social work practitioners understand that policy affects service delivery, and they actively engage in policy practice. Social workers know the history and current structures of social policies and services, the role of policy in service delivery, and the role of practice in policy development. Social workers

- Analyze, formulate, and advocate for policies that advance social well-being;
- Collaborate with colleagues and clients for effective policy action.

EDUCATIONAL POLICY 2.1.9

Respond to contexts that shape practice.

Social workers are informed, resourceful, and proactive in responding to evolving organizational, community, and societal contexts at all levels of practice. Social workers recognize that the context of practice is dynamic, and use knowledge and skill to respond proactively. Social workers

- Continuously discover, appraise, and attend to changing locales, populations, scientific and technological developments, and emerging societal trends to provide relevant services;
- Provide leadership in promoting sustainable changes in service delivery and practice to improve the quality of social services.

Educational Policy 2.1.10(a)–(d)—Engage, assess, intervene, and evaluate with individuals, families, groups, organizations, and communities.

Professional practice involves the dynamic and interactive processes of engagement, assessment, intervention, and evaluation at multiple levels. Social workers have the knowledge and skills to practice with individuals, families, groups, organizations, and communities. Practice knowledge includes identifying, analyzing, and implementing evidence-based interventions designed to achieve client goals; using research and technological advances; evaluating program outcomes and practice effectiveness; developing, analyzing, advocating, and providing leadership for policies and services; and promoting social and economic justice.

Educational Policy 2.1.10(a)—Engagement.

Social workers

- Substantively and affectively prepare for action with individuals, families, groups, organizations, and communities;
- Use empathy and other interpersonal skills;
- Develop a mutually agreed-on focus of work and desired outcomes.

Educational Policy 2.1.10(b)—Assessment.

Social workers

- Collect, organize, and interpret client data;
- Assess client strengths and limitations;

- Develop mutually agreed-on intervention goals and objectives;
- Select appropriate intervention strategies.

Educational Policy 2.1.10(c)—Intervention.

Social workers

- Initiate actions to achieve organizational goals;
- Implement prevention interventions that enhance client capacities;
- Help clients resolve problems;
- Negotiate, mediate, and advocate for clients;
- Facilitate transitions and endings.

Educational Policy 2.1.10(d)—Evaluation.

Social workers critically analyze, monitor, and evaluate interventions.

Chapter	Professional identity	Ethical practice	Critical thinking	Diversity in practice	Human rights & justice	Research-based practice	Human behavior	Practice contexts	Engage, assess, intervene, evaluate
1	X	X	X		X	X			
2		X	X	X		X		X	
3						X	X		X
4			X			X			X
5	X		X			X		X	X
6			X			X		X	X
7	X		X			X		X	X
8			X			X		X	X
9	X		X			X		X	X
10			X			X		X	X
11	X		X			X		X	X
12			X			X		X	X
13	X		X			X		X	X
14			X			X		X	X
15	X		X			X		X	X
16			X	X	X	X			X
17			X	X	X	X			X
Total Chapters	7	2	16	3	3	17	1	12	15

CHAPTER 1

Introduction

MENTAL ILLNESS is a serious public health problem that
goes largely unrecognized by many Americans. In the United
States, it is the number one cause of disability and costs
approximately $79 billion each year due to loss of produc-
tivity, incarcerations, and mortality-related expenses (New
Freedom Commission on Mental Health, 2003). Mental
illness is more common than other illnesses such as
cancer, heart disease, or diabetes. Anyone, regardless
of age, gender, race, ethnicity, and socioeconomic
status, can experience a mental health problem. In
fact, most of us will experience a mental health
problem sometime in our lives. At the same
time, the majority of Americans (nearly
70%) will not seek any form of treatment
for their own mental health problem or
their children's mental health problem because they do not recognize
it as a serious problem or
because of the stigma that
can be attached to mental

illness (U.S. Department of Health and Human Services, 2009). Mental health problems left untreated can cause long-lasting problems. For children, these problems can interfere with their socioemotional and cognitive development (Institute of Medicine, 2009). Left untreated, these problems can follow them into adulthood. Research has found that nearly 50 percent of adults experiencing a mental illness begin experiencing symptoms as early as age fourteen and as many as 75 percent experience symptoms by age twenty (Kessler et al., 2005). The sad realization is that mental health problems can and should be treated. With proper treatment, a person can experience recovery and lead a full, happy, healthy life.

An increased focus on mental illness has occurred over the past several years due to mass shootings reported in the media. Unfortunately, this media coverage has also increased the stigma associated with mental illness. One needs to keep in perspective that the vast majority of persons with a mental health problem will never harm themselves or others (Phillips, 2012; see also Satcher, 2000). They are far more likely to be victims of a crime than perpetrators. The focus on the mass shootings has been both a vehicle to open the conversation on mental illness and treatment and a means of increasing the stigma. Being knowledgeable about mental health problems and how to identify them and understanding that treatment can be effective are important factors in reducing mental health stigma and increasing treatment seeking for those in need.

It has been well established that at any given time, an estimated 1 in 5 children is experiencing some form of mental illness, with 1 in 10 children suffering from a serious mental illness resulting in significant impairments across all aspects of their lives (Center for Behavioral Health Statistics and Quality, 2011). The proportion of children with serious emotional or behavioral problems in the child welfare and juvenile justice systems is even higher than the national average (Carney & Buttell, 2003; U.S. General Accounting Office, 2003). Fortunately, our knowledge of factors contributing to children's mental health problems has increased, as has the development of treatments found to be effective in ameliorating these problems.

The objective of *Understanding the Mental Health Problems of Children and Adolescents* is to provide a practical guide for social workers in promoting positive mental health in youth from a bio-socio-ecological systems perspective. Social workers will gain an understanding of the scope of mental health issues in youth to include definitions, etiology, and evidence-based treatments. Further, social workers will understand the importance of partnering with youth and caregivers, addressing issues from a strengths perspective, and engaging in culturally sensitive practice. Social workers will want to take this work and apply it actively in their everyday work with clients.

The mental health community is continually updating current knowledge in the field. On the date that this book was sent to the publisher, the National Institute of Mental Health published a report, *Five Major Mental Disorders Share Same Genes*, demonstrating that knowledge is fluid and that what we are presenting in this book is the knowledge base at this moment in time. As reported, the largest study yet into genetics and mental health (Cross-Disorder Group, 2013) "reveals that the five most common disorders—autism, attention deficit hyperactivity disorder, bipolar disease, schizophrenia, and major depression—all share similar genetic components. . . . The results suggest that a rethink in how these disorders are defined might be in order. Rather than focusing on symptoms, which can be attributed to one or more disorder, physicians could one day start to rely on specific gene mutations or biologic pathways to make a formal diagnosis" (National Institute of Mental Health, 2013).

Research advances in behavioral science and neuroscience have greatly improved our knowledge and understanding of mental illness. Magnetic resonance imaging (MRI) has allowed researchers to gain greater knowledge of brain development and changes in the brain related to mental illness. Brain research has given practitioners the evidence base that they have long been describing in behavioral, emotional, and psychological terms. This knowledge base will continue to grow and influence treatment.

MENTAL ILLNESS

Mental illnesses are among the most pressing public health issues today. Mental illness can be categorized into two distinct types, situational and serious and persistent. Situational mental illnesses are usually temporary. They can arise in anyone who is experiencing some type of severe stress and has trouble coping with the situation. Serious and persistent mental illnesses are the result of certain psychological, biological, genetic, or environmental conditions. Serious and persistent mental illness can include behavioral disorders such as oppositional defiant disorder and conduct disorder or brain disorders such as schizophrenia, schizoaffective disorders, major depression, and bipolar disorder. Serious mental illness can be treated and managed effectively if an individual has access to a combination of medication, supportive counseling, and community support services, including education and vocational training. With proper treatment, people experiencing mental illness can return to normal, productive lives. However, stigma remains a major barrier, discouraging individuals from seeking help. Again, nearly two-thirds of all people with a diagnosable mental health disorder do not seek treatment (U.S. Department of Health and Human Services, 2009). Analysis of consumer and public input has identified stigma as one of seven major categories to be addressed for mental health transformation (Center for Behavioral Health Statistics and Quality, 2011).

In 2001, as part of his New Freedom Initiative, President George W. Bush directed members of the New Freedom Commission to study problems in the mental health system and make recommendations. In 2003, the New Freedom Commission reported children's mental health to be a public health crisis in the United States, noting the existence of many barriers that impede children from receiving appropriate mental health care. These barriers include a fragmented service delivery system, stigma and stigmatizing behaviors against persons experiencing a mental illness, financial barriers, a lag between discovery of effective treatments and their implementation, lack of early identification and intervention, and lack of adequately trained mental health professionals. Although we know more about the serious consequences of untreated mental health problems and effective treatments than we did in 2003, many of these problems continue to exist. Untreated and inadequately treated youth are ending up in the child welfare or juvenile justice systems. Approximately 36 percent of youth in the juvenile system nationally become involved due to inadequate or unavailable mental health services, and thousands of families each year are forced to relinquish custody of their children in order to receive mental health treatment (Carney & Buttell, 2003; U.S. General Accounting Office, 2003).

Stigmatizing attitudes and behaviors toward individuals with mental health problems present multiple barriers that have severe consequences for quality of life. The New Freedom Commission identified stigma as one of three main obstacles that impede individuals with mental illness from receiving appropriate treatment. The consequences of stigma include delays in treatment, challenges to self-esteem, social isolation, discrimination, and lost opportunities in such areas as housing and employment. In addition to mental health stigma, the lack of treatments available to persons in the community is a huge barrier. The research on effective treatments for children with mental health problems has increased dramatically over the past several years, but many children lack access to these treatments for many reasons. Although there has been an increase in knowledge of effective treatments, child welfare, juvenile justice, and community mental health systems have experienced a lag in adoption and implementation of evidence-based practices (EBPs) and program/treatments (EBTs) due to financial constraints, lack of infrastructure, and controversy around EBTs (Burns & Hoagwood, 2002; Hoagwood, 2001).

Compounding the challenge of embracing EBP in these child-serving sectors are organizational structures that are not amenable to adhering to the fidelity of empirically supported treatments (Hoagwood, 2001; Huang, Hepburn, & Espiritu, 2003; Jensen, Weersing, Hoagwood, & Goldman, 2005). Evidence-based practices and treatments have specified practices and processes (fidelity) that must be followed in order to realize the positive outcomes that are reported in the empirical literature (Fixsen, Naoom, Blase, Friedman, & Wallace, 2005). As a result, a vulnerable population of children in high need of these treatments does not receive them or does not receive them as developed. Failure to provide effective treatments to this population results in higher costs to systems. High-risk youth and families reenter these systems over and over or youth end up being placed in more restrictive settings outside of their homes and communities. Not providing effective treatment can also result in long-term costs to these systems as untreated youth often carry their problems into adulthood, resulting in lost wages, repeating the cycle of abuse, or incarceration, to name a few of the possible consequences (Anderson, Wright, Kelley, & Koorman, 2008).

DIAGNOSING AND THE DIAGNOSTIC AND STATISTICAL MANUAL

In this book the signs and symptoms of the most commonly diagnosed mental health disorders of childhood and adolescence will be reviewed, followed by a discussion of treatment. A person is diagnosed with a mental health problem or illness by a professional trained and authorized to make diagnoses following an extensive face-to-face evaluation. Psychiatrists, licensed professional counselors, licensed marriage and family counselors, and licensed clinical social workers are all professionals with the training and authority to diagnose mental health problems. During the face-to-face assessment, the clinician must determine if a person meets the diagnostic criteria for a specific mental health disorder as specified in the International Classification of Diseases (ICD) developed by the World Health Organization or the *Diagnostic and Statistical Manual of Mental Disorders (DSM)* published by the American Psychiatric Association. Most clinicians in the United States use the *DSM* for diagnosing mental health problems.

The diagnostic codes of mental health disorders in the *DSM* are linked to the diagnostic codes in ICD-9-CM (clinical modification) and ICD-10-CM (World Health Organization, 1992). The ICD is the official coding system approved by the Health Insurance Portability and Accountability Act (HIPAA). Insurance companies require a psychiatric evaluation and assignment of a mental health ICD diagnostic code for authorization and reimbursement for services rendered. The ICD is currently in its tenth revision and the eleventh revision (ICD-11) is underway.

Comparison of the *DSM-IV* and the *DSM-5*

The first version of the *DSM* (*DSM-1*) was published in 1952. Since its inception, the *DSM* has gone through several revisions and is currently in its fifth edition (American Psychiatric Association, 2013). The *DSM* provides a common language among mental health professionals for making accurate diagnoses. It helps guide treatment planning and it provides a common language for mental health researchers. The diagnostic criteria for each mental health disorder indicate what specific symptoms must be present for each diagnosis and for how long they must have occurred. Exclusionary criteria are also specified for each disorder. Across all disorders, other plausible causes such as a medical condition, substance abuse, or other mental health conditions must be ruled out as the cause of the problems. This can be difficult as people often experience co-occurring problems.

Prior to the *DSM-5*, the last major revision of the *DSM*, *DSM-IV*, occurred in 1994 (American Psychiatric Association); when this book was begun, the current version of the *DSM* was the *DSM-IV-TR* (American Psychiatric Association, 2000). The *DSM-IV-TR* used a multi-axial system for diagnosis. Clinicians rated different aspects of a mental health diagnosis across five axes. Axis I included all the major diagnostic categories with the exception of personality disorders and mental retardation. Diagnoses discussed in this book, formerly known as axis I diagnoses for children and adolescents, include depression, anxiety, bipolar disorder, attention deficit hyperactivity disorder, oppositional defiant disorder, and schizophrenia. On axis II, a clinician recorded personality disorders (e.g., borderline, histrionic, or narcissistic personality disorder) and/or mental retardation if applicable. If the clinician did not have enough information about axis II, he or she deferred a diagnosis until more information was available. It was not common practice to diagnose a young person with a personality disorder because of developmental issues and the stigma that can follow a person with that diagnosis. General medical conditions including acute medical conditions and physical disorders that may aggravate an existing mental health condition or may present similarly to a mental health disorder were recorded on axis III. Axis IV is where a clinician reported psychosocial and environmental factors that contribute to the mental health disorder. The *DSM-IV* groups these factors into the following categories:

- Problems with primary support group
- Problems related to the social environment
- Educational problems
- Occupational problems
- Housing problems
- Economic problems
- Problems with access to health care services
- Problems related to interaction with the legal system/crime
- Other psychosocial and environmental problems

On axis V, clinicians provided a subjective rating of daily functioning across social, occupational, and psychological functioning on the Global Assessment of Functioning for adults or rated general functioning of children and adolescents on the Children's Global Assessment Scale. Both scales are scored from 1 to 100, with higher scores indicating a higher level of functioning and lower scores indicating severe impairment resulting from a mental health problem. Scores of 0 indicate insufficient information to provide a score.

The *DSM-5* has undergone significant changes from the *DSM-IV*. The overall structure of the manual has been changed to order disorders based on shared similarities of symptom characteristics. This structural change further aligns the *DSM* with the World Health Organization's ICD-11.

Another significant change is that the *DSM-5* no longer documents diagnoses across the five axes. Axes I, II, and III are combined. Separate notations are used for recording what were formerly axes IV and V. The new structure of the *DSM-5* is based on evidence that the boundaries between different mental health disorders are less clear-cut than once thought, as many of the disorders share similar symptoms and similar genetic and environmental risk factors. New disorders have been added to *DSM-5* or moved from Appendix B of the *DSM-IV-TR* to be included as a diagnosis. *Specifiers* are used throughout the *DSM-5* to document important factors that may have played a role in the development of a disorder. The new structure of the *DMS-5* takes a lifespan focus by presenting diagnoses on a continuum based on the stage in the life cycle where the disorder most commonly manifests, beginning with disorders thought to begin early in the developmental processes and ending with those that manifest in late adulthood.

The first section of the *DSM-5* presents neurodevelopmental disorders, which are those disorders that manifest during childhood development. Examples of neurodevelopmental disorders include intellectual disabilities, autism spectrum disorder, communication disorders, motor disorders, learning disorders, and attention deficit hyperactivity disorder. The next four sections focus on schizophrenia and psychotic disorders, bipolar and related disorders, depressive disorders, and anxiety disorders respectively. Obsessive-compulsive disorders and related disorders comprise a new section that includes disorders characterized by preoccupations and rituals. These disorders were included in anxiety disorders in the *DSM-IV-TR*. The final section addresses trauma- and stress-related disorders.

Throughout this book, significant changes in the classification of a disorder from *DSM-IV-TR* to *DSM-5* will be discussed as relative to each chapter.

WHAT EVERY CHILD NEEDS FOR GOOD MENTAL HEALTH

Although mental illness/mental health problems are the focus of this book, it is important to recognize factors important to good mental health. The ingredients needed for a child to develop good mental health are well recognized. Children need to receive unconditional love as well as encouragement, guidance, and appropriate discipline from their caregivers. Providing boundaries for youth along with encouragement and guidance allows them to safely explore their world and develop positive self-esteem and self-confidence. Children and adolescents need to live in an environment that is both physically and emotionally safe. Finally, to develop socially, they need to have relationships with peers near their own age with whom they can play, interact, and develop relationships.

Trauma, chaotic homes, violence, neglect, parental mental health problems, biology, and child temperament can all be contributing factors to the development of serious emotional and behavioral problems (Institute of Medicine, 2009). The United States has focused on crisis intervention rather than early identification and intervention. Evidence shows that we can make greater impact on mental health problems by identifying and treating them early on.

Although this book addresses diagnosing mental health disorders and discusses evidence-based practices and interventions specific to each disorder, it is important to consider the individual. The phrase "I am not my mental illness" was used in an anti-stigma campaign commissioned by the Mental Health Connection (MHC) of Tarrant County, a community collaborative of public and private agencies, individuals experiencing mental health problems, and their families with the intent to revolutionize mental health services in their community. It is important to interact with every person as an individual and not to make assumptions based on what we see on the surface or based on a label given as a diagnosis. Although providing a diagnosis gives us a common language, the diagnosis should not be the only thing we see. Each person is unique and has strengths. Mental illness is one aspect of a person's life; it is not his or her entire life. Clinical practice should consider each person's uniqueness, strengths, determination, and needs, as well as the climate that surrounds him or her (ecological system model). As you will see in some of the case scenarios provided throughout the book, things are not always as they appear at first.

Although we talk about a singular diagnosis, many persons experience more than one mental health problem at a time. This can make determining the appropriate treatment challenging and involve sound clinical judgment. Although there are interventions found to be effective in treating nearly all mental health problems, the improvements are often modest and they are not effective for everyone. In addition, there are many barriers to accessing empirically supported treatments in the community; cost to implement and resistance from providers are among the major impediments. As you read this book, please keep these things in mind and critically assess your role in the provision of services to youth and families.

REFERENCES

American Psychiatric Association. (1994). *Diagnostic and statistical manual of mental disorders* (4th ed.). Washington, DC: Author.

American Psychiatric Association. (2000). *Diagnostic and statistical manual of mental disorders* (4th ed., text revision). Washington, DC: Author.

American Psychiatric Association. (2013). *Diagnostic and statistical manual of mental disorders* (5th ed.). Washington, DC: Author.

Anderson, J. A., Wright, E. R., Kelley, K., & Koorman, H. (2008). Patterns of clinical functioning over time for young people served in a system of care. *Journal of Emotional and Behavioral Disorders, 16*, 90–104.

Burns, B. J., & Hoagwood, K. (Eds.). (2002). *Community treatment for youth: Evidence-based interventions for severe emotional and behavioral disorders*. New York: Oxford University Press.

Carney, M. M., & Buttell, F. (2003). Reducing juvenile recidivism: Evaluating the wrap-around services model. *Research on Social Work Practice, 13*, 551–568.

Center for Behavioral Health Statistics and Quality. (2011). *Results from the 2010 National Survey on Drug Use and Health: Summary of national findings* (HHS Publication No. SMA 11-4658, NSDUH Series H-41). Rockville, MD: Substance Abuse and Mental Health Services Administration.

Cross-Disorder Group of the Psychiatric Genomics Consortium. (2013). Identification of risk loci with shared effects on five major psychiatric disorders: A genome-wide analysis. *The Lancet, 381*(9875), 1371–1379. doi:10.1016/S0140-6736(12)62129-1

Fixsen, D. L., Naoom, S. F., Blase, K. A., Friedman, R. M., & Wallace, F. (2005). *Implementation research: A synthesis of the literature* (FMHI Publication 231). Tampa, FL: University of South Florida, Louis de la Parte Florida Mental Health Institute, The National Implementation Research Network. Retrieved from http://nirn.fpg .unc.edu/sites/nirn.fpg.unc.edu/files/resources/NIRN-MonographFull-01-2005.pdf

Hoagwood, K. (2001). Evidence-based practice in children's mental health services: What do we know? Why aren't we putting it to use? *Emotional and Behavioral Disorders in Youth*, Fall, 84–87.

Huang, L. N., Hepburn, K. S., & Espiritu, R. C. (2003). To be or not to be . . . evidence-based? *Data Matters, 6*, 1–3.

Institute of Medicine. (2009). *Preventing mental, emotional, and behavioral disorders among young people: Progress and possibilities*. M. E. O'Connell, T. Boat, & K. E. Warner (Eds.). Washington, DC: National Academies Press.

Jensen, P. S., Weersing, R., Hoagwood, K. E., & Goldman, E. (2005). What is the evidence for evidence-based treatments? A hard look at our soft underbelly. *Mental Health Services Research, 7*, 53–74.

Kessler, R. C., Berglund, P., Demler, O., Jin, R., Merikangas, K. R., & Walters, E. E. (2005). Lifetime prevalence and age-of-onset distributions of DSM-IV disorders in the National Comorbidity Survey Replication. *Archives of General Psychiatry, 62*, 593–602.

National Institute of Mental Health. (2013). *Five major mental disorders share the same genes*. Retrieved from http://www.nimh.nih.gov/news/science-news/2013/five-major -mental-disorders-share-the-same-genes.shtml

New Freedom Commission on Mental Health. (2003). *Achieving the promise: Transforming mental health care in America*. Final report (DHHS Publication No. SMA-03-3832). Rockville, MD: Department of Health and Human Services.

Phillips, R. T. M. (2012). Health law: Predicting the risk of future dangerousness. *Virtual Mentor, 14*, 472–476.

Satcher, D. S. (2000). Mental health: A report of the Surgeon General—Executive summary. *Public Health Reports, 115*, 89–101.

U.S. Department of Health and Human Services. (2009). *Substance Abuse and Mental Health Services Administration: Justification of estimates for Appropriations Committees*. Rockville, MD: U.S. Department of Health and Human Services, Substance Abuse and Mental Health Services Administration, Center for Mental Health Services, National Institutes of Health, National Institute of Mental Health. Retrieved from http://beta.samhsa.gov/sites/default/files/samhsa_cj2009.pdf

U.S. General Accounting Office. (2003). *Child welfare and juvenile justice: Federal agencies could play a stronger role in helping states reduce the number of children placed solely to obtain mental health services*. Retrieved from http://www.gao.gov /highlights/d03397high.pdf

World Health Organization. (1992). *The ICD-10 classification of mental and behavioural disorders: Clinical descriptions and diagnostic guidelines*. Geneva: Author.

CHAPTER 2

Framework for Understanding and Treating Mental Health Problems

AS AN OVERARCHING FRAMEWORK, this book empha-
sizes the importance of five components when working with
children and families with mental health problems: the ecological systems model, systems of care, evidence-based
practices and programs, cultural sensitivity, and engagement and strengths-based practices.

ECOLOGICAL SYSTEMS MODEL

The ecological systems model provides the wide
lens for understanding the multiple layers within
the family system. It goes beyond assessing
relations and interactions between the
parent and youth to look at the effects of
all systems in the youth's environment.
According to the theory, a developing individual is affected by the
environments in which he or
she resides as well as by settings in which he or she is

not present (Bronfenbrenner, 1979). In effect, the individual affects those environments. A person cannot be studied without including his or her environment in the analysis. The components of ecological systems are the microsystems, mesosystems, exosystems, and macrosystems. The *microsystem* in which a person resides (e.g., a child's family) has the most influence. The *mesosystem* includes settings outside the microsystem in which an individual participates. The child's school and peer group are examples of mesosystems. Individuals are members of multiple social groups, or mesosystems, at the same time.

A setting such as the workplace of a child's parent is an *exosystem* to a child. A child may not have direct contact with the workplace of a parent, yet the workplace affects the child, and the child affects the workplace. For instance, a parent who is overstressed by pressures of employment may lack energy to provide a child adequate attention and care. On the other hand, a parent may perform poorly at work due to stress resulting from difficult issues with a child or may miss days at work due to the child's mental health problems.

People continuously attempt to adapt to their environment. They either try to improve the fit between themselves and their environment or they try to sustain a good fit (Germain & Bloom, 1999). Understanding the adaptations a child has developed to fit in his or her environment is a key factor to treating the child. It is also important to identify factors in the ecological system model that either facilitate or impede adaptation. Individuals are usually able to adapt to conventional environments, but they may struggle to adapt during stressful times or in conditions in which they have special needs or limitations.

As life events occur, people deal with them either positively or negatively, depending on their perception of the event. The way in which the person views an event will allow him or her to either cope with it and achieve a successful resolution or prevent him or her from coping with it, leading to an unsuccessful resolution. The response of the individual will affect both the environment and the individual. Successful resolution leads to personal development and/or environmental change.

In order to understand a life event, one must fully consider all aspects of the person-environment, including all of the systems and subsystems that affect adaptation. These systems and subsystems include a person's cognitive, biological, affective, and behavioral structures in addition to subsystems of the environment. The relationship between people and environments in which they are embedded is dynamic. A circular relationship exists in that a change in one area of the system will affect all other levels of the system. Changes in the system will thus affect the individual. We either adapt to our environment or seek to change it. An example of *reciprocation and exchange* can be seen when a child or adolescent is placed in a residential treatment facility to receive mental health treatment aimed at improving problem behaviors. Typically, the child or adolescent fights against the new environment and resists change, yet eventually he or she adapts and problem behaviors improve. If the family does not make changes in the home environment aimed at sustaining the child's or adolescent's behavior changes, the problem behaviors will eventually return. Each element of the system affects another.

Mental health problems develop from multilayered interactions between the youth and the environment. A therapist must consider the dimensions of human temperament and personality in addition to the external environment, culture, and socioeconomic existence of the youth and family. Effective intervention in a youth's mental health problems requires assessment of personal factors (biological, genetic, and psychological) as well as factors across the entire ecology to understand what sustains or diminishes the problem behavior. How does the youth normally react to stressful situations? Does the youth currently have the tools needed to be successful socially and emotionally? Is there a familial genetic predisposition that puts the youth at a higher risk for a certain problem? These are just some of the questions to examine.

The logic of the ecological system model is one of the strengths of the model, allowing it to take into account a larger relationship than linear models. It allows one to see factors in the environment that may either impede or provide an opportunity for a person's growth. The ecological system model allows for a more complete assessment of a situation and provides more information than general systems theory because it encourages the assessment of interactions between systems. Thus, it expands a social worker's thinking as to the causes of problems and allows interventions focused on the total picture rather than only the personal factors.

SYSTEMS OF CARE

Systems of care, initially proposed in the mid-1980s, are a family-centered, strengths-based service delivery model (Stroul & Friedman, 1996). Within systems of care, community-based supports and services are organized to meet the challenges of children with serious mental health needs and their families. In 1993, the systems of care movement was enhanced by the development of the Comprehensive Community Mental Health Services for Children and Their Families Program (Center for Mental Health Services, 2006), the most significant federal investment in children's mental health to that date, to address the critical problems experienced by youth with serious emotional disturbances and their families. Referrals to systems of care come from a range of child service agencies including schools, child welfare, state mental health, juvenile justice, and parole and probation. Systems of care seek to remove the silos among juvenile justice, mental health, and child welfare systems and empower families, not only to make decisions about their own treatment, but also to affect policy and practice. Developing systems of care is a national movement. A key philosophical underpinning of systems of care is that youth and families are equal partners with equal voice working alongside professionals in the treatment process. Family empowerment has been noted to be a key mediator in improving children's mental health. Treating the youth and family as an equal partner in all decision making is a major paradigm shift for child welfare, juvenile justice, and mental health systems.

In an effort to provide effective care for children with serious emotional disturbances consistent with the values and principles of systems of care, many states and communities have adopted the wraparound process of mental health care and management (Bruns & Suter, 2010; Burns, Goldman, Faw, & Burchard, 1999; Furman & Jackson, 2002; Suter & Bruns, 2009). Wraparound has been described as a promising practice for treating youth experiencing severe emotional or behavioral problems. It has been identified as both a philosophy and a process of providing supports and services to youth with serious emotional disturbances and their families and a tool for implementing systems of care. In wraparound, a child and family team is developed based on the desires of the family. Team members may include family members, friends, schoolteachers, pastors, mental health professionals, or any other persons important to the family. A wraparound facilitator guides the team to develop, implement, and monitor a comprehensive service plan. The service plan, developed from the individual needs, strengths, and desires of the family, draws on both formal resources (including evidence-based practices and programs) and informal services and community supports aimed at improving the mental health of the child and keeping him or her in the community.

EVIDENCE-BASED PRACTICES AND EVIDENCE-BASED PROGRAMS

The literature is increasingly emphasizing the importance of *evidence-based practice* (EBP) and *evidence-based program or treatment* (EBT). At the same time, there is both confusion and controversy about these terms. There is confusion about what they mean. There is also controversy about what level of science exists to designate treatments and interventions as evidence based. How is evidence determined? Many question where clinical experience fits into EBT. So, just exactly what is meant by these terms? These are important issues to understand as we begin to incorporate EBT and EBP into practice with families and children.

The terms *evidence-based practice* and *evidence-based treatment* are often used interchangeably; however, they do not refer to the same things. In mental health treatment, an evidence-based practice refers to the provision of clinical practices or techniques that are based on the best available research evidence to achieve the best positive outcomes. The American Psychological Association defines evidence-based practice as "the integration of the best available research with clinical expertise in the context of patient characteristics, culture, and preferences" (American Psychological Association Presidential Task Force, 2006).

An evidence-based program (treatment) refers to a multicomponent intervention based on a combination of empirically supported evidence-based practices (core components) that have been highly researched and found to be effective in meeting targeted outcomes. These multicomponent programs are based on the theoretical underpinnings of the ecological system model, in conjunction with other theoretical perspectives such as cognitive, behavioral, and social learning theories. Some EBTs follow a more theoretical approach to treatment based on the individual needs of a youth and family, whereas others utilize a manualized approach following a specific protocol. In some instances, mental health providers have been reluctant to use many of the programs or treatments, particularly those that are manualized, feeling that they take their clinical skill and perspective out of the equation. Although most manualized approaches encourage adherence to the treatment, many also encourage integration of the individual clinical skills and uniqueness of the treatment provider into the treatment.

The profession of social work began incorporating EBP models into the professional literature around 2003. Today, the literature is increasingly emphasizing its importance. Although there has been increased emphasis in the literature on the importance of EBT and early identification and treatment of youth with mental health problems, there is a lack of social workers trained in mental health issues of children and EBP and/or EBT. Evidence-based interventions and practices are not being taught in university settings or in community child service settings. Social workers in the workforce are uninformed about EBP/EBT and mental health issues of childhood because of their lack of access to relevant training. A possible contributor to the lack of social worker training is the controversy surrounding EBP and EBT. In particular, most, if not all, EBT models require focused training and ongoing clinical supervision from the developer or organization.

The National Association of Social Workers (NASW) has adopted an approach to EBP that is inclusive of knowledge based on research, clinical skills, and individual determination of those receiving services. Our knowledge is constantly growing and practices are adapted or new treatments emerge based on the best available research. The onus is on all of us to contribute to the knowledge, to understand what the knowledge is telling us, and to understand the gaps in our knowledge. In past years, excluding empirical evidence from clinical treatment has resulted in practitioners providing treatments that not only lack evidence of effectiveness, but in some instances have been found to be ineffective or even harmful. Examples of harmful interventions include boot camps for youth experiencing acting out behaviors and *rebirthing* for children diagnosed with reactive attachment disorder. Empirical research indicates that sending youth to boot camp to manage acting out behaviors can further exacerbate their problems, for example by increasing anger at caregivers for putting them into harsh conditions away from friends and family, not acknowledging their underlying need for and providing mental health treatment, and exposing them to other youth with similar or worse problems. At least two children have died from rebirthing, in which they are put into a fetal position and swaddled in a wrap such as a blanket to represent the womb. Therapists then simulate labor contractions by putting pressure on the womb and the child fights his or her way out as a way to bond with the caregiver.

Throughout this book, we will refer to and differentiate among existing EBPs and EBTs for different mental health disorders. However, we should remember not to ignore our own clinical judgment, the strengths and needs of the people we work with, or the evidence base as it exists at each moment. Similarly, we should continue to pursue new knowledge and incorporate it into treatment.

CULTURAL SENSITIVITY

The disproportionality of minority children, especially African American children, in both the child welfare and criminal justice systems has been well documented over the years. Overrepresentation of minority children and families refers to the difference between their representation at a particular time in the child welfare or juvenile justice system compared to their representation in the general population during the same time period. Minority children account for 15 percent of the U.S. child population; however, they represent 37 percent of the children who are involved in the child welfare system (Wulczyn & Lery, 2007).

Compounding the issue of the disproportionality of minority children in the child welfare and juvenile justice systems is the percentage of youth in these systems needing mental health care. In the United States, nearly one million children each year come into contact with the child welfare system because they are victims of child abuse or neglect. Many are at high risk of mental health problems resulting from maltreatment, removal from their homes, and/or the trauma of investigation and intervention by child welfare. The percentages of children with clinically significant emotional or behavioral problems in both systems have been found to be much higher than in the general population. Nationally, it is estimated that 50 to 80 percent of youth investigated for child maltreatment experience significant mental health problems. In the juvenile justice system, estimates of youths experiencing mental health problems are as high as 65 or 70 percent.

The disparity in the number of minority youth accessing mental health care, the quality of care they receive, and their representation in mental health research has been highly acknowledged in the literature. This disparity is mirrored in the child welfare and juvenile justice systems as well. Minority youth receive fewer services such as birth family visits, developmental and psychological assessments, worker contacts, treatment plans, and mental health services than Caucasian youth.

ENGAGEMENT AND STRENGTHS-BASED PRACTICE

Many would argue that it is the relationship with the social worker rather than the provision of an EBP or EBT that helps clients reach their goals. Youth and family engagement and strengths-focused problem solving are critical ingredients in the helping process of social work. Most or all social workers would probably agree. On paper and in theory, these concepts sound good. What do they really mean and how does engagement and strengths-focused problem solving look in practice?

Although we as social workers agree with the values and ethics of social work, we often find ourselves telling our clients what is best for them and what the consequences will be if they choose to ignore our warnings. This can be particularly true of social workers working in juvenile justice, child welfare, and community mental health settings. We get our college degree and go into the workforce, armed with the values of our profession, with the desire to make a difference in others' lives. In the new work environment, we may start to take on the culture of the agency in which we work, which is made up of persons from many backgrounds and degree programs with varying views. Our intent is good, but we may lose our vision somewhere along the way.

It is important to revisit the practice of social work and our own role and practice. Although research is very clear on the correlation of high levels of engagement and positive outcomes, it is difficult to break out of patterns developed within the culture of an agency. We begin to use phrases such as those stating that the client is "resistant to change" or "resistant to participating in treatment." We even use the social work value of *self-determination* as a reason to discharge youth and families from services, claiming that they have a right to make the choices they make and a right to experience the consequences of those choices. Engaging families requires us to thoroughly examine the situation when a family is not engaging. Lack of engagement is unlikely to occur because a caregiver wants to keep harming his or her child or the youth wants to end up in a detention facility. Problems with engagement can be caused by one or a culmination of situations with the family, the individual worker, and the agency.

One possible reason for lack of engagement is that family members have worked with several persons in the helping profession and have not received the help they need. They may feel as if you are just another person in a string of people who will not be able to meet their needs. Past experience may have discouraged their belief that things can get better. Alternatively, the family may be experiencing such a large amount of stress or chaos that thinking about trying to add anything into the mix seems daunting, even if you tell them that it will change things in the future. Due to stereotypes in the media and other venues, many people believe that the only role and purpose of social workers is to take away their children. Other reasons may include the family's lack of transportation, long working hours, or focus on daily necessities such as providing food to eat.

Your own characteristics or situations and/or those of the agency may block engagement. It is easy to get bogged down with heavy caseloads, documentation requirements, and agency rules and regulations. Such distractions may cause us to miss the factors that prevent us from engaging with families. The stress in our lives can engulf us and leave us without the energy needed to engage with families. Engagement takes work on the front end, but makes the middle and end of our journey with youth and families much more productive and satisfying.

What other reasons can you think of that may be barriers to engagement? Think through the question and write down as many reasons as you can. Next, think about and write down some tactics you as the social worker can use to overcome each barrier. Be creative in your tactics. Sometimes the smallest of gestures will go far in building relationships. Remember that every individual and family you work with will have unique situations. It is incumbent upon you as the social worker to determine the issues that are relevant in each situation. The more things you can identify as possible barriers, the more prepared you will be when you work with families.

Exercise: Barriers and Solutions to Engagement

Barrier 1:

Possible Solution(s):

Barrier 2:

Possible Solution(s):

Barrier 3:

Possible Solution(s):

Barrier 4:

Possible Solution(s):

Case Scenarios

Following are some real life examples of things social workers have done to engage families. As you read these scenarios, think about the barriers and solutions you identified. Do these scenarios spark any other ideas?

Jenny is a social worker at a community mental health center. She is having difficulty meeting with a mother to get paperwork signed so that she can start working with Jon, her six-year-old son. The mother canceled one meeting and was not home when Jenny arrived for a second meeting. When Jenny was able to talk to the mother on the phone later that day, the mother sounded frustrated. She vented about missing the second meeting because she had taken the bus to the food stamp office. She had to change buses twice to get there and she missed the second bus. By the time she finally arrived at the food stamp office, she had missed her appointment and had to reschedule for the next week. This left her without the needed food stamps so she took the bus to a food pantry to get some food, but she wasn't able to get enough to last until her next appointment because she couldn't carry much. Recognizing the situation that the mother was in and the frustration she was experiencing, Jenny offered to drive her to the food pantry the next day and to drive her to the food stamp office for the next appointment. On the way to the food pantry, Jenny was able to chat with the mother. After she took the mother to the food pantry, they sat down and completed the paperwork needed to get Jon into services.

In another situation, a social worker, Otis, was assigned to work with Nguyen and his family, who had been given the option of participating in a diversionary program or sending Nguyen to a detention center. The family chose the program. As part of the program, they were to meet with Otis a couple of times every week. However, both parents worked two jobs and did not have time to meet with Otis. They worked together in the evening cleaning offices. They made Nguyen go to work with them in the evening to keep him out of trouble. Otis asked if he could meet with the family while they cleaned the offices. Otis even helped clean offices so the parents had some time to sit and work with him.

Both Jenny and Otis could have said that the family would not or could not meet with them and discharged the family rather than trying to seek a solution. This would have meant that Jon would not have received the needed treatment and Nguyen would have been locked up in detention. Other social workers have done things such as offering to bring pizza to the family for dinner so that they could meet.

REFERENCES

American Psychological Association Presidential Task Force on Evidence-based Practice. (2006). Evidence-based practice in psychology. *American Psychologist, 61,* 271–285.

Bronfenbrenner, U. (1979). *The ecology of human development: Experiments by nature and design.* Cambridge, MA: Harvard University Press.

Bruns, E. J., & Suter, J. C. (2010). Summary of the wraparound evidence-base. In E. J. Bruns & J. S. Walker (Eds.), *The resource guide to wraparound.* Portland, OR: National Wraparound Initiative.

Burns, B. J., Goldman, S. K., Faw, L., & Burchard, J. D. (1999). The wraparound evidence base. In B. J. Burns & S. K. Goldman (Eds.), *Promising practices in wraparound for children with severe emotional disorders and their families* (pp. 77–95). Rockville, MD: Center for Mental Health Services.

Center for Mental Health Services. (2006). *Annual report to Congress on the evaluation of the Comprehensive Community Mental Health Services for Children and Their Families Program, 2001.* Atlanta, GA: ORC Macro.

Furman, R., & Jackson, R. (2002). Wrap-around services: An analysis of community-based mental health services for children. *Journal of Child and Adolescent Psychiatric Nursing, 15,* 124–131.

Germain, C. B., & Bloom, M. (1999). *Human behavior in the social environment: An ecological view* (2nd ed.). New York: Columbia University Press.

Stroul, B., & Friedman, R. (1996). The system of care concept and philosophy. In B. Stroul (Ed.), *Children's mental health: Creating systems of care in a changing society.* Baltimore, MD: Paul H. Brookes.

Suter, J. C., & Bruns, E. J. (2009). Effectiveness of the wraparound process for children with emotional and behavioral disorders: A meta-analysis. *Clinical Child Family Psychological Review*, *12*, 336–351.

Wulczyn, F., & Lery, B. (2007). *Racial disparity in foster care admissions*. Chicago: Chapin Hall Center for Children at the University of Chicago.

CHAPTER 3

Overview of Child and Youth Development

THIS BOOK focuses on youth from six to eighteen years of age. This chapter is a summary and brief overview of the major developmental milestones and characteristics of the children and youth in this age range. It will exclude infancy-toddlerhood and early childhood and begin with children entering middle childhood. (For a full overview, see Scannapieco & Connell-Carrick, 2005.)

MIDDLE CHILDHOOD

There is great diversity among children and families in the United States, but generally we view middle childhood as a time for education, team play, social activities, and other forms of leisure. Development takes place within the domains of physical, social, and cognitive dimensions (see Table 3.1). Each of these domains will be presented separately, but they occur in an interactive, dynamic fashion.

Table 3.1. Middle childhood healthy development (6–11 years of age)

Psychodynamic

Freud

Latency:
- Sexual instincts decrease.
- The superego develops further with more influence from peer relationships and less from family.
- Children put their energy into activities, such as school and sports, and their sexual needs become inert.

Erickson

Industry versus inferiority:
- Children busily try to master the activities valued by their culture.
- The positive resolution of this crisis is the development of industry whereby children feel competent and productive in their ability.
- Children continue to master new skills and continue to develop social skills and friendships.
- The negative resolution of inferiority manifests as children feel unable to do anything well.

Social

- Children engage in organized games with rules.
- Social cognition develops; children begin to understand their social world.
- Peer groups become increasingly important, which helps develop self-concept and self-competence.
- Acceptance by peer groups is valued, but personal friendships are more important.
- Perspective taking increases.
- Children develop a more realistic level of self-competence and self-esteem.
- Peer interaction becomes more pro-social.

Cognitive (Piaget)

Concrete operational stage: Reasoning and logical thought begin.
- Children are able to conserve and organize objects into hierarchies.
- Children have the ability to interpret experiences objectively rather than intuitively.
- Children understand logical principles and apply them to concrete situations, not hypothetical situations.
- Children understand identity, reversibility, seriation, and spatial reasoning.
- Children still fail to have abstract reasoning.
- Improvement in memory occurs, including an ability to remember facts over a period of days.
- Memory strategies improve: rehearsal, organization, and elaboration.
- Vocabulary at age six should be 10,000 words.
- Selective attention develops, which becomes important for school and learning.
- Metacognition develops, which is the ability to evaluate a cognitive task to determine whether it is difficult or not.
- Code switching in language emerges: formal and informal codes are used in communicating with adults and friends, respectively.

Table 3.1. (Continued)

Physical

- Children grow more slowly.
- Children have slimmer bodies with stronger muscles.
- Gross motor skills of running, jumping, batting, and kicking are performed more quickly and with better coordination.
- Reaction time improves in relation to cognitive development.
- Flexibility, hand-eye coordination, balance, force, agility, and judgment of movement improve.
- Fine motor development improves (e.g., building models or weaving on small looms).
- Printing improves from large letters to smaller letters.
- Drawing improves with two-dimensional shapes, depth, and converging lines.

Middle childhood extends from six to eleven years of age. During this time, children enter formal school, and academics and social relationships become increasingly important. Overall, the primary developmental task of middle childhood is the acquisition of new skills—cognitive, social, and physical—and children have school as a new forum for exploration. During what are sometimes called the *school years*, children not only learn the foundations of math, reading, writing, and science, but they also practice their social skills with their peer group.

Expected Development over Developmental Domains

Psychodynamic Theories

Freud's Psychosexual Stages of Development. Freud's fourth stage of psychosexual development is called the *latency stage* and occurs between six and eleven years of age. During the latency period, sexual instincts subside and become dormant. Instead of putting their energy into psychosexual activities, children focus on more conservative tasks including school and sports. In previous stages, children were influenced primarily by their parents. The latency stage exposes children to formal education and the opportunities that it offers; thus, children are influenced by their peers, their teachers, and the leaders of their organized activities. Their superegos continue to develop as a result of external influences.

Erickson's Psychosocial Stages of Development. During middle childhood, the psychosocial conflict proposed by Erickson is that of *industry versus inferiority*.

During the school years, children try to master new cognitive and physical activities. They learn to cooperate, share, and problem solve with other children, and as a result, a sense of industry arises. Children with a resolution of industry feel competent at accomplishing tasks alone and with others. However, when children do not acquire the ability to work with others or they have negative experiences in completing solitary activities, they develop a sense of inferiority. Not all children have the same opportunities, and some may be more vulnerable due to poverty, community violence, and school inequities. In these cases, children may have had negative experiences when attempting tasks. Children who do not resolve the psychosocial crisis with inferiority feel incompetent.

Physical Development

Children from six to eleven years of age grow more slowly than before; on average they grow two to three inches and gain three to five pounds per year. Girls experience their adolescent growth spurt before boys, which may result in girls growing quickly in both height and weight toward the end of this period. Children's bodies become slimmer, and the lower portions of their bodies grow faster. Children may grow out of their jeans faster than their jackets as their legs grow longer. During middle childhood children commonly complain of growing pains, or nighttime aches and pains that occur as their muscles grow and adapt to their changing bodies. They should continue to receive regular medical and dental checkups, as primary teeth are gradually replaced by permanent teeth.

Motor Development

During middle childhood children continue both their fine and gross motor development. Gross motor development improves, with children being able to successfully play organized activities and group sports with rules. Throwing, swimming, and climbing improve. These skills are demonstrated with better coordination and more quickly than ever before. Children also become better at bicycle riding, swimming, and ballet, which require good coordination.

Children from six to eleven years of age have greater flexibility, balance, agility, and force. The combination of their gross motor developmental changes and their cognitive changes allows children to play sports well; they make quick decisions as they develop skilled movements. As an example, school-aged children play baseball with a strong, quick, and flexible swing, and they demonstrate the ability to abide by the rules.

Fine motor development also continues throughout middle childhood. Children in this period should begin to print letters and learn cursive handwriting. They should be able to print and write stories, and their written words become clearer with age. Similarly, drawing improves so that by the end of this period children can make two- and three-dimensional drawings with attention to detail, depth, and lines. However, girls develop fine motor skills, including drawing and handwriting, faster than boys and girls outperform boys on gross motor skills that require balance and agility, such as jumping. On the other hand, boys outperform girls in throwing and kicking, primarily due to environmental influences and practice rather than genetics.

Cognitive Development

According to Piaget's theory of cognitive development, children enter the middle childhood years during the second stage—*preoperational thought*—and finish this phase at the third stage—*concrete operational thought*. This stage is marked by the child's ability to distinguish reality from perception. During this period, children are capable of more logical thought; they are able to process operations that require compliance with logical rules. For example, children can pass conservation tasks in which they must focus on more than one aspect of the task in order to solve the problem appropriately. In the early childhood stage, if a child were asked to choose between two beakers with equal amounts of liquid but different shapes, he or she would choose the taller beaker. In this stage, the child would recognize that the beaker being taller does not mean that it has more liquid, but that the shape of the glass affects the appearance of the liquid.

Children between six and eleven years of age experience an improvement in memory. Children can retrieve stored information for days or longer. They also demonstrate selective attention, whereby they are able to screen out distractions and focus on the important information. For example, during class the ten-year-old will be able to pay attention to the teacher while ignoring and forgetting disruptions from nearby classmates. Thus, the child selectively tunes in to the important information being presented by the teacher. Children also begin to use strategies to improve their memory, such as rehearsal, elaboration, and organization. Rehearsal, or repeating information over and over in an attempt to remember it, begins early in this period. Elaboration involves creating a shared meaning between two or more pieces of information that are not in the same category.

Children in middle childhood focus on both physical attributes and inner traits of a person. A child may describe a person physically, but add that the person is dull or kind, referring to inner traits. Children at this stage are capable of *perspective taking*, or the ability and capacity to understand what others may be thinking or feeling. They consider the perspective of another person in relation to their own thoughts and those of others, and this helps them to understand consequences, such as getting in trouble or offending a friend. Acquiring a more mature level of perspective taking is important because without it children risk offending peers and further isolating themselves from social relationships.

Social Development

As indicated by Erickson's psychosocial theory, the acquisition of feelings of self-competence is the major developmental task during this period. Children become more complicated social beings as they enter school and new opportunities arise. Changes in self-esteem, self-concept, and peer relationships occur.

As children mature, they begin to become more interested in peer relationships and they become more independent. Their relationship with their parents is still important; however, school friendships and lifelong friendships emerge. Playing together is no longer the essential measure of friendship, and qualities such as trust and loyalty begin to define true friendships. After children are able to identify friends through more mature characteristics, they use these friendships to practice conflict resolution and joint problem solving. Consistent with their understanding of internal characteristics and their gains in cognitive development, children also make social comparisons; they begin to more realistically appraise their own behavior and skills compared to those of their peers.

Children understand their proficiency relative to that of another peer, which is influenced by their cognitive development and their expanding social worlds. Friendships during middle childhood tend to be gender segregated and occur around shared activities.

With more realistic self-appraisal, children adjust their self-esteem to fit their perceptions and evaluations of self. As a result, self-esteem tends to drop during the first years of elementary school, but increases again from fourth to sixth grade. By age six, children have separated their self-esteem into three different domains: academic, social, and physical. They are able to appraise themselves in each of these three areas; for example, a child may have high academic self-esteem but less social self-esteem.

Aggression is still common in middle childhood, but to a lesser degree than in the previous developmental period. By middle childhood, children have learned the cultural and social rules that govern acceptable behavior. Society also expects children to be more able to control their anger by the time they reach middle childhood. At any rate, girls and boys tend to express their anger in different ways. Girls tend to use more *relational aggression*—nonphysical aggression aimed at damaging another's self-esteem or peer relationships. For example, a girl may try to ostracize another child or belittle her among friends. On the other hand, boys tend to use more physical force to express anger. However, both sexes exhibit increased aggression aimed at retaliating against someone who has injured them, called *retaliatory aggression*. Although peers accept retaliatory aggression, it is not accepted by parents, teachers, and coaches.

Peer groups also become an important component of middle childhood. Although true friendships are valued, acceptance by peer groups is also sought. Peer groups tend to be informal, with their own language and vocabulary, and they have a special identity. The peer group has collective goals, leadership, and loyalty. Often it can take the form of a group that engages in organized activities, such as a soccer or basketball team. Another example of the influence of peer groups will be discussed in the section on adolescence. Children switch their language when speaking with adults and peers to reflect the formality of the situation.

ADOLESCENCE

Adolescence is a transitional time between childhood and emerging adulthood characterized by profound biological, cognitive, and social changes. According to much of the recent developmental theory, it begins at age twelve and ends roughly around age twenty-four (Sokol, 2009). Although current developmental theory may extend adolescence until age twenty, this chapter will focus on adolescence from twelve to eighteen, when a child becomes a legal adult in the eyes of the court.

Adolescence is marked by changes in physical, cognitive, and social development (see Table 3.2). The most obvious changes are those that are visible, whereas mood and social changes tend to be the most difficult for adolescents and others to understand. Teens may become sexually active with peers and they may become pregnant. They are exploring their own identities, trying to find out

Table 3.2. Adolescent development characteristics

Psychodynamic

Freud

Genital:
- With puberty sexual impulses reemerge.
- The genitals are the focus of pleasure and the young person seeks sexual stimulation and satisfaction.

Erickson

Identity versus role confusion:
- Adolescents try to discover a self-identity through political, social, sexual, and career identities.
- The primary job of adolescents is to establish intimate ties with others.
- Adolescents who have had previous negative resolutions have difficulty establishing ties to others and are confused about their identity and roles.

Social

- Parent-adolescent conflict and moodiness increase, but vary depending upon age, gender, and culture.
- Friendships become even more important and influential.
- Peer groups are important and based on similar interests and values.
- Loyalty and intimacy are crucial to friendships.
- Peer pressure has both constructive and destructive abilities.
- Sexual and romantic relationships begin.

Cognitive (Piaget)

Formal operational stage:
- Adolescents have the ability for abstract thought and scientific reasoning.
- Hypothetical reasoning is possible, and problems are approached with logic and reasoning.
- Adolescents can think about ideas rather than only concrete events.
- As a result, ethics and social and moral issues become even more interesting.
- With increases in hypothetical and abstract thought, adolescents have better ability to argue.
- Metacognition and emotional regulation are enhanced.
- With age, adolescents become better at decision making and planning.
- Adolescent egocentrism develops whereby the adolescent focuses on himself or herself, believing that his or her thoughts, beliefs, and feelings are unique experiences.
- The *invincibility fable* emerges: a way of thinking in which adolescents feel immune to the dangers of their behaviors.

Physical

- Puberty begins.
- For girls, puberty sparks the onset of breast growth, initial pubic hair, peak growth spurt, widening of hips, and first menstrual period.
- For boys, puberty sparks the onset of pubic hair, growth of testes and penis, first ejaculation, growth spurt, voice deepening, and beard development.
- The average age of menarche is 12.5 years.
- For girls, motor performance peaks and then levels off.
- The average age of spermarche is 13.
- Adolescents may have sexual intercourse.

who they are and what they really believe. They are spending more time away from home with friends, who become even more influential and more important than before.

Expected Development over Developmental Domains

Psychodynamic Theories

Freud's Psychosexual Stages of Development. Freud's sixth stage of psychosexual development is the *genital stage*, which begins in adolescence and lasts through adulthood. The adolescent's primary focus is on sexual pleasure and stimulation, coinciding with the onset of puberty. The major developmental task during this period is to achieve mature sexual intimacy. Because much of Freud's genital stage is focused on sexuality, it will be further expanded upon in the section on physical development.

Erickson's Psychosocial Stages of Development. Erickson proposed that the major psychosocial crisis of adolescence is *identity versus role confusion.* A major psychosocial task is the development of a self-identity while maintaining some form of group ideals. Teens who resolve this crisis positively leave with a set of self-chosen values, goals, morals, and political ideology. They are not confused about what role to play in various aspects of their life; they may have explored other identities during adolescence, and by the end of this period, they have settled on a self-chosen one. Individuals who negatively resolve this crisis appear directionless, confused, and shallow. They will be unprepared for the daunting task of adulthood. It is important to mention that previous developmental thought was that the search for an identity was an *identity crisis*, but current thought is that this is not a crisis at all (Grotevant, 1998). It may be difficult for loved ones to adapt to the new changes, ideas, and thoughts of the adolescent, but the teen is not in crisis, but rather in search of an identity.

Adolescents do not initially arrive at a decision; instead they often search for an identity throughout this period. Four identity patterns emerge during adolescence when teens move in and out of various identities before deciding on one (Marcia, 1966):

- *Identity achievement.* Adolescents who have attained identity achievement have positively resolved the psychosocial crisis of deciding upon an identity. These adolescents have explored alternatives and have a set of self-chosen values, goals, and morals. They have critically looked at their belief systems and accepted some parts of them while rejecting others to settle on self-chosen ideals. A sense of psychological peace settles with these teens.

- *Identity moratorium.* Identity moratorium is characterized by a delay in identity achievement. This individual is not making firm commitments to an identity, but rather is exploring various thoughts and activities. Attending college is often thought of as a socially constructed moratorium in which students can try different identities and behaviors until they decide what is appropriate for them.
- *Identity foreclosure.* Identity foreclosure occurs when adolescents fail to question traditional values; they do not take the time to explore various alternatives, but prematurely decide on a set of values and goals that others have chosen for them. An example of this is a teen who becomes a preacher because his father and grandfather were both preachers, and this decision is expected of him.
- *Identity diffusion.* Identity diffusion occurs when adolescents are directionless. They are not in search of a self, goals, or values and they have not committed to any. Many teens find the task of exploring their identity daunting and overwhelming and therefore fail to do so. They appear apathetic and may even have difficulty doing tasks that require thinking about the future. They may fail to commit in friendship or romantic relationships.

Adolescence is marked by decisions concerning an individual's life: college or vocational school, work, personal values, goals, and aspirations. It is important to understand that identity discovery is culture based. In cultures in which there is virtually universal adhesion to social norms and roles, the transition of adolescence into adulthood is relatively short and easy. When few options exist, deciding on an identity is a short and quick decision. This is a time of great self-exploration for many teens, and it is an important one. Teens who are able to fully explore the challenges ahead are prepared for adulthood.

Physical Development

Physical change is greater than at any time other than infancy (Rathus, 2003). The physical changes of puberty are the most obvious signs of adolescence. During puberty the reproductive system matures. Within a few years, a child's body is transformed into an adult body. The boy's testes release large quantities of testosterone, which result in facial and body hair, voice deepening, muscle development, and overall growth in height and weight. The female ovaries release large quantities of estrogen and the adrenal gland releases the adrenal hormone, resulting in breast development, menstruation, body shape changes, and growth in height. Both sexes undergo a growth spurt, a rapid gain in height; however, girls encounter their growth spurt before boys. Eventually, however, boys catch up to girls and tend to be taller and ultimately heavier. Testosterone and estrogen are released in both boys and girls, but each sex receives a larger amount of one.

Sexual maturation is one of the most important aspects of puberty. From middle childhood, the body changes into a reproductive system. The average age of menarche (first menstruation) for girls is 12.5, and the average age for spermarche (first ejaculation) is 13 for males. Although the signs of puberty seem quite sudden, the hormonal changes that underlie puberty begin much earlier. By the time the results of the hormonal changes are evident, they have been underway for some time. In addition to sexual maturation, there are skeletal system changes so that adolescents increase in height; their joints develop further, allowing better coordination. The muscular system continues to develop so that adolescents become stronger and have a high level of physical performance.

One of the ways scientists have searched for the causes of mental illness is by studying the development of the brain from birth to adulthood. New technologies have enabled them to track the growth of the brain and to study the connections between brain function, development, and behavior. This research has turned up some surprises, among them the discovery of striking changes taking place during the teen years (National Institute of Mental Health, 2012).

Contrary to earlier thoughts, the adolescent brain continues to grow and develop (Johnson, Blum, & Giedd, 2009). Recent research by Johnson and colleagues reveals the development of the frontal lobes during adolescence and indicates that they may not be fully developed until age twenty-five. The frontal lobes direct the executive functions of planning, memory, and impulse control. One interpretation of these findings is that in teens the parts of the brain involved in keeping emotional, impulsive responses in check are still reaching maturity. This may help to explain adolescents' appetite for novelty and tendency to act on impulse without regard for risk.

Although much is being learned about the adolescent brain, it is not yet possible to know to what extent a particular behavior or ability is the result of a feature of brain structure. Changes in the brain take place in the context of many other factors, such as genetics, childhood experiences, family, friends, community, and culture.

Cognitive Development

Adolescence is marked by changes in thinking. Piaget named the time period from age eleven or twelve to adulthood the formal operational stage of cognitive development, which is the final stage of his developmental theory. The formal operational stage of cognitive development is characterized by increased cognition in many areas. Adolescents can think about possibilities rather than only about concrete events as in the previous stage (concrete operational stage) and they can think abstractly. They can mentally solve hypothetical problems, which is a marked difference from the previous stage. One consequence of this new thinking, however, is that teens may think they know the answers to complex and multidimensional problems. Sometimes they become critical of their parents and their parents' choices. For example, a teen may think that she knows how to have a good marriage and criticize her mother for what she did wrong to ruin her own marriage. It is noteworthy that not all individuals reach the formal operational stage or all of the cognitive gains in it; even those who go to college do not pass all formal operational tests.

Adolescents are able to think about how things could be rather than merely how they are. Adolescent thinking is characterized by hypothetical thought. The teenager may think hypothetically about what life will be like if she or he stays close to home for college or goes far away. Sometimes this new capacity for thinking frustrates parents because teens are constantly trying out their new ideas of politics, education, and relationships, for example. They may make judgments about morality, and they often challenge traditional ideas.

Adolescents are also capable of deductive reasoning, and this is one of the primary reasons why courses such as geometry are taught in high school rather than earlier. Teens are able to reason about if-then statements. They can systematically solve problems by starting with a premise and testing hypotheses. Adolescent science projects often reflect their deductive thinking capabilities.

Adolescent thinking is characterized by egocentric thoughts. Teens tend to overestimate their significance among friends and groups and feel that other people are keenly interested in them. They may feel that they have an imaginary audience, that everyone is watching them. This helps explain why they will spend a large amount of time getting ready, choosing an outfit, or fixing their hair. Alternatively, a teen may not want to go to a particular store for fear that someone might see her there, even though the person seeing her would also be in the store. With this elevated sense of importance, teens may imagine their own lives as ultimately being magical and heroic. For example, a teen may feel that all violence is wrong regardless of the reason because all individuals are created equal and deserve respect. She may feel that, if she could only tell the U.S. attorney general about this, he would understand this wrongdoing and change policies regarding violence in our country.

Adolescents become more aware during adolescence—they become more aware of themselves, others, and their place in the world. This combination of egocentrism and thinking about possibilities rather than realities makes adolescence a time when teens feel that they have explored all rational solutions to a problem, but rarely have done so. The egocentrism in their thinking influences their ability to consistently make well-informed decisions.

Social Development

In addition to Erickson's psychosocial crises, many other developmental activities affect social development in adolescence. Even though the adolescent years can be trying for parents, who are struggling to understand the changes in their child, children with strong attachments to their parents are able to weather the tasks of adolescence better than those with poor attachments, and these attachments will remain strong during adolescence despite the influence of peers. Strong attachments to parents are predictive of high academic achievement and good peer relationships (Black & McCartney, 1997). Similarly, teens who have good relationships with their parents are less likely to use drugs, in both adolescence and adulthood. However, teens and parents tend to bicker and argue more at home during adolescence. They fight about petty things such as hair, clothing, and cleaning. Teens often try to obtain adult privileges during adolescence and seek privacy. Although this can be a trying time, it is developmentally appropriate as teens try to embrace tasks of adulthood with new cognitive skills and access to social functions.

One of the primary tasks of adolescence is the discovery of self. Self-esteem often changes in adolescence. Adolescents have generally high levels of self-esteem, but this varies from individual to individual. Some factors associated with a decline in self-esteem include school transition, late physical development, poor academic performance, and drug use. Children whose parents use an authoritative style of parenting have generally higher levels of self-esteem. Research also shows that both boys and girls who have an androgynous or masculine self-concept/identity have higher self-esteem (Burnett, Anderson, & Heppner, 1995) although cross-cultural research suggests that this may not be true for all cultures (Lobel, Slone, & Winch, 1997).

Peer relationships become important during middle childhood, but they become even more so during adolescence. Friendships take on new functions. Intimacy and loyalty become important. Adolescents search for psychological closeness to their friends; they tend to feel that nobody understands them (Rathus, 2003), and their friends provide a forum to feel understood. Adolescent friendships are also characterized by loyalty: sticking up for one another becomes important in the cohesion of friendships.

Another component of friendships is self-disclosure, in which teens tell each other personal things about themselves to be held in confidence among friends. Such intimacy among friends is not seen in middle school children, but is an important part of adolescent friendships. Friends also provide social support to one another, and this helps ease coping with physical and emotional challenges. Adolescents get to know their friends better as people, including their dreams and goals, rather than just as playmates. They try to preserve friendships because of their shared intimacy and loyalty, and they try to resolve conflicts with their close friends as opposed to just ending the friendship.

Peer groups and cliques also form among teen friends with similar characteristics. Peer groups become more prevalent in adolescence. Teens gather in groups with shared liking of activities and often thoughts. The peer group is structured, often around shared family background, socioeconomic status, and attitudes. Peer pressure frequently has a negative connotation, but it is not always bad. Peer groups often pressure friends to abstain from drugs or smoking and can serve many positive functions. Special peer groups, often referred to as cliques, such as the brains, jocks, druggies, and popular kids, form during school. Cliques frequently have shared language (also seen in middle childhood), dress, and behaviors or activities. Association with peer groups and cliques changes over time, however. Toward late adolescence teens are less concerned with cliques because, if they have attained identity achievement, they have less need for crowd or peer influence with their identity. At any rate, peer groups help share adolescent thinking and exploration of identities.

One of the challenges of adolescent relationships is the development of romantic relationships. Friendships in middle childhood are primarily among same-sex friends, but adolescent friendships change to include members of the opposite sex. Not all different-sex friendships evolve into romantic relationships, but most teens have a conceptual understanding of being in love with another. As in same-sex friendships, girls tend to seek psychological closeness with members of the opposite sex through self-disclosure, whereas boys seek this less. Romantic relationships tend to be intense but short lived. Adolescence is a time of sexual exploration, although the degree of this is influenced by peers, family structure, and religious upbringing.

Although romantic relationship development is important in adolescence, so is the decision about one's individual sexual development. By the time they complete high school, the majority of males and females are likely to have engaged in sexual intercourse (Miller, Levin, Whitaker, & Xu, 1998). Social factors are good predictors of the likelihood of sexual activity, including low socioeconomic status, lack of adult supervision, and familial acceptance of dating and sex, as well as child sexual abuse (Herrenkohl, Herrenkohl, Egolf, & Russo, 1998).

Much of our developmental theories focus on heterosexual sexual development, but recent research has also looked at the unique challenges of gay and lesbian adolescents. Gay and lesbian adolescents face unique challenges compared to their heterosexual counterparts, including whether or not to disclose their sexual orientation and how to handle the response from peers and family. Furthermore, gay and lesbian teens have a smaller dating pool because many teens are still discovering their sexuality. Many teens do not label themselves as gay or lesbian, but rather remain undecided in adolescence as they are discovering their sexual and personal identities. At any rate, both heterosexual and gay and lesbian teens face many of the same insecurities and challenges. Males in both groups are more likely to drink alcohol, females in both groups are more likely to diet, and both groups are likely to fear rejection from their partners. However, many adolescent lesbians and gays feel different from their heterosexual peers (Wormer, Wells, & Boes, 2000).

THE BRAIN

Throughout this book, brain research targeted to each mental health disorder or problem will be discussed. Knowledge gained through research examining brain development and changes that occur related to mental health disorders and trauma helps us understand what the child is experiencing biologically and its impact on development. In social work practice with children, it is important to be aware of the changes in brain function that occur with all mental health disorders. The size of a child's brain is 80 percent the size of an adult brain by age two and 90 percent by age five. It is extremely important for social workers and others working with children who are experiencing social, emotional, and behavioral problems to conduct thorough bio-socio-ecological assessments prior to treatment.

In order to understand the role of the brain in mental illness, it is important to have a basic understanding of how the brain works. The brain is made up of three basic units: the forebrain, consisting of the cerebrum and hidden structures of the inner brain; midbrain, consisting of the uppermost part of the brainstem; and hindbrain, consisting of the spinal cord, the brainstem, and cerebellum (National Institutes of Health, 2014). Within these units are specialized areas working together to mediate different functions of the body.

The regions of the brain consist of grey and white matter. Grey matter consists mostly of the cell bodies of nerve cells, called neurons. These neurons communicate with billions of synapses and stimulate sacs that release the chemicals known as neurotransmitters into the synapses. Neurotransmitters attach to the receptors of other cells and can either change the properties of the new cells or transmit to another cell if the cell is also a neuron. These neurotransmitters seem to play significant roles in mental illnesses.

Grey matter is associated with intelligence. It is responsible for gathering information from sensory organs and passing the information to where it needs to go. White matter, which consists of axons of nerve cells and myelin, makes up other parts of the brain and is responsible for helping grey matter communicate to the rest of the body. Grey and white matter continue to transform through early adulthood.

The brain develops from less complex structures, such as the brainstem (lower part of the brain that connects the spinal cord to the cerebral hemispheres), to the more complex structures of the reticular activating system (RAS) located within the brainstem and one of the most important structures in the brain. The RAS is made up of billions of neurons and glial cells organized into systems with the purpose of sensing, processing, storing, perceiving, and acting on both the internal and external environments. Neurons are the raw material of the brain, and glial cells are supportive cells located in the brain and spinal cord, also known as the central nervous system.

The RAS is involved in arousal, anxiety, and modulation of limbic and cortical processing. The limbic system, located in the cerebrum part of the brain, has been found to be responsible for regulating emotions and formation of memories. It is also responsible for affect regulation and the development of attachment. It consists of key structures such as the hypothalamus, hippocampus, amygdala, and locus coeruleus. The hypothalamus regulates our ability to control anger and aggressive behavior. It also regulates things such as hunger, ability to feel pleasure, sexual satisfaction, and the autonomic nervous system that controls our arousal responses and the physical aspects connected to our arousal responses such as breathing, pulse rate, and blood pressure.

The cognitive aspects of memory are stored in the hippocampus. The hippocampus plays a major role in memory and learning and in activities of the autonomic nervous system and the neuroendocrine system. It is located near the cortex and lower diencephalic (back of the forebrain) areas of the brain. It is believed to play a significant role in the pathophysiology of anxiety and panic attacks due to excess noradrenergic influences from the locus coeruleus. It is further believed that the hippocampus plays a role in the behavioral inhibitory system that acts to stop socially inappropriate behavior. Repeated stress inhibits development of neurons (specialized cells that conduct electrochemical impulses) and causes atrophy of dendrites (short branched fibers where nerve impulses are generated). This results in functional problems of memory and learning.

The amygdala is located in the cerebral hemispheres of the brain. The emotional aspects of memory are stored in the amygdala. The amygdala is the most sensitive brain structure for the emergence of kindling, which causes spontaneous electric discharges. Kindling results in long-term alterations in neuronal excitability, which can affect behavior. The amygdala plays a key role in emotional memory processing, interpreting and integrating emotional functions. It also plays a role in fear conditioning and control of aggressive oral and sexual behavior. Key to orchestrating a response to areas of the brain, the amygdala is involved in motor, autonomic nervous system, and neuroendocrine areas of the central nervous system.

The locus coeruleus, part of the catecholamine system, functions as a general regulator for noradrenergic tone and activity. The ventral tegmental nucleus is also part of the catecholamine system. The catecholamine system plays a critical role in regulating arousal; vigilance; affect; and stress, behavioral irritability, locomotion, attention, sleep, and startle responses. The locus coeruleus is a bilateral nucleus of norepinephrine-containing neurons that regulates the sympathetic nervous system and activities of the autonomic system and hypothalamic-pituitary-adrenal axis. If incoming sensory information is threatening, the locus coeruleus increases its activity and releases norepinephrine (a neurotransmitter) into key areas of the brain and body. When norepinephrine is released, changes occur in heart rate, blood pressure, respiratory rate, muscle tone, and glucose mobilization, resulting in the release of the potentially brain-damaging hormones adrenocorticotropin and cortisol. The ventral tegmental nucleus also releases norepinephrine when activated by acute stress.

When subjected to extreme stress, the body responds by releasing hormones such as cortisol or adrenaline, which have been shown to damage brain cells, disrupt homeostasis, impair memory, and affect the sympathetic nervous and endocrine systems. The changes in these systems thus effect changes in other body systems, such as the cardiovascular, respiratory, and muscular systems. Acute stress resulting in neurophysiologic activation is reversible; however, these changes can be irreversible in cases of stress at high levels of frequency, duration, or intensity. Brain research on mental health disorders focuses on the amygdala, hippocampus, and prefrontal cortex regions of the brain.

REFERENCES

Black, K., & McCartney, K. (1997). Adolescent females' security with parents predicts the quality of peer interactions. *Social Development, 6*, 91–110.

Burnett, J., Anderson, W., & Heppner, P. (1995). Gender roles and self-esteem: A consideration of environmental factors. *Journal of Counseling and Development, 73*, 323–326.

Grotevant, H. D. (1998). Adolescent development in family contexts. In N. Eisenberg (Vol. Ed.) & W. Damon (Series Ed.), *Handbook of child psychology: Social, emotional, and personality development* (Vol. 3, pp. 1097–1149). New York: Wiley.

Herrenkohl, E., Herrenkohl, R., Egolf, B., & Russo, M. (1998). The relationship between early maltreatment and teenage parenthood. *Journal of Adolescence, 21*, 291–303.

Johnson, S., Blum, R., & Giedd, J. (2009). Adolescent maturity and the brain: The promise and pitfalls of neuroscience research in adolescent health policy. *Journal of Adolescent Health, 45*, 216–221.

Lobel, T., Slone, M., & Winch, G. (1997). Masculinity, popularity, and self-esteem among Israeli preadolescent girls. *Sex Roles, 36*, 385–408.

Marcia, J. E. (1966). Development and validation of ego-identity status. *Journal of Personality and Social Psychology, 3*, 551–558.

Miller, K. S., Levin, M. L., Whitaker, D. J., & Xu, X. (1998). Patterns of condom use among adolescents: The impact of mother-adolescent communication. *American Journal of Public Health, 88*, 1542–1544.

National Institute of Mental Health. (2012). *The teen brain: Still under construction* (NIH Publication No. 11–4929). Retrieved from http://www.nimh.nih.gov/health/publica tions/the-teen-brain-still-under-construction/index.shtml

National Institutes of Health. (2014). *Brain basics: Know your brain* (NIH Publication No. 11–3440a). Bethesda, MD: Author. Retrieved from http://www.ninds.nih.gov /disorders/brain_basics/know_your_brain.htm

Rathus, S. A. (2003). *Voyages in childhood*. Belmont, CA: Wadsworth, Thompson Learning.

Scannapieco, M., & Connell-Carrick, K. (2005). *Understanding child maltreatment: An ecological and developmental perspective*. New York: Oxford University Press.

Sokol, J. T. (2009). Identity development throughout the lifetime: An examination of Eriksonian theory. *Graduate Journal of Counseling Psychology, 1*, article 14. Retrieved from http://epublications.marquette.edu/gjcp/vol1/iss2/14

Wormer, K., Wells, J., & Boes, M. (2000). *Social work with lesbians, gays, and bisexuals: A strengths perspective*. Boston: Allyn Bacon.

CHAPTER 4

Depressive Disorders

FEELING SAD OR DOWN is common for all children and
teens. Situational depression due to a best friend moving
away, loss of a pet, or making a bad grade can be expected.
Clinical depression goes beyond situational depression.
Persistent feelings of sadness and changes in behavior
such as decreased interest in favorite activities, isolation,
changes in sleeping or eating habits, and decreased
grades can be an indication of a more serious problem (American Psychiatric Association, 2013).
When feelings of sadness persist and a child or
teenager has difficulty functioning in daily life,
the situation needs to be taken seriously and
not ignored.

Children do experience serious
depression. The reality is that as many
as 1 in 33 children experience clinical depression, meaning a serious
depression that significantly
interferes with their lives
(Merikangas et al., 2010).

Merikangas and colleagues report that, as youth reach adolescence, these numbers change to as many as 1 in 8 experiencing serious depression. When depression is ignored, it can lead to academic underachievement, social isolation, difficult relationships with family and friends, increased risk of drug and alcohol abuse, and increased risk for suicide (National Institute of Mental Health, n.d.-a, n.d.-b).

CAUSES OF DEPRESSION

The causes of depression in children and teenagers are similar to the causes of depression in adults. It is believed that depression is caused by a combination of risk factors such as genetic vulnerability, biochemical disturbances in the brain, environment, poor coping or problem-solving skills, and family history (National Institute of Mental Health, n.d.-a). Children with a family history of depression are three times more likely to experience depression than children without such a family history (Tsuang & Faraone, 1990).

Stressful life events such as the death of a caregiver, divorce, or a chaotic living environment can be triggers to serious depression. Other triggers may include moving to a new school, failing a grade, or being bullied. Children and teenagers who have experienced abuse, neglect, a chronic illness, or other traumatic event are at a higher risk of developing serious depression. Youth in the child welfare and juvenile justice systems have been found to experience higher rates of serious depression than other youth.

Brain research on the biology of depression has focused on the limbic system; hypothalamus; and three neurotransmitters: serotonin, norepinephrine, and dopamine (Krishnan et al., 2004). Researchers are also studying genes that they believe make some people susceptible to depression and the hormone cortisol that has been found to be elevated in depressed persons (Tsuang & Faraone, 1990).

DEPRESSION AND THE BRAIN

The limbic system is made up of many structures that regulate functions in the body (Kandel, Schwartz, & Jessell, 2000). The amygdala and hippocampus, two structures of the limbic system, are involved in regulating emotion. The hypothalamus regulates anger, aggression, hunger, ability to feel pleasure, sexual arousal, and stress response.

When we think, feel, or react, neurotransmitters send messages through the limbic system. Serotonin, norepinephrine, and dopamine are the neurotransmitters that transmit messages in the limbic system and hypothalamus. Researchers have found a connection between these three neurotransmitters and clinical depression, but just how they are connected is not quite known (National Institute of Mental Health, n.d.-a). What is known is that levels of these neurotransmitters are altered in persons with depression. Researchers are not sure which comes first. Either a person becomes depressed, resulting in changes in the levels of the serotonin, norepinephrine, or dopamine, or changes in the levels of the neurotransmitters cause depression. Researchers continue to study the causes of depression in an effort to better understand the underlying causes and to develop more effective treatments.

SIGNS AND SYMPTOMS OF DEPRESSION

There are many signs suggesting that a child or adolescent is experiencing depression and is in need of an evaluation by a mental health professional. Changes in sleeping and eating patterns can be a sign of depression. The youth may begin sleeping too much or having difficulty falling or staying asleep and/or experience significant weight gain or loss. One may notice changes in cognitions, behavior, and personality. Irrational beliefs can lead a once confident youth to become highly sensitive to rejection or failure. These feelings are often not based in the reality of the situation. A once happy youth may exhibit frequent tearfulness or sadness. Both children and adolescents experiencing depression may exhibit self-destructive behavior or overreact emotionally to what may seem to be small things to those around them. A decrease in self-esteem is usually evident. It is common for youth experiencing depression to begin talking about themselves in self-deprecating or negative ways. When these youth look in the mirror, they may see a distorted version of themselves. They may perceive themselves to be ugly or fat.

Changes in motivation and energy level are also very common. The youth may seem to move more slowly, talk more slowly, or not seem interested in anything. A classic sign of depression in youth is a decreased interest in things once enjoyed and a decreased interest in hanging out with friends, such as when the youth who once enjoyed playing basketball after school or going to the mall to hang out with friends stops engaging in these social activities and begins spending more and more time isolated in his or her room. It is common for depressed teenagers to begin listening to music about death or aggressive subjects or to draw pictures or write about subjects that include death, suicide, or morbid subjects. In children, signs of depression can often be seen in their play. Their play may involve aggression that is directed toward themselves or others, or it may persistently involve themes that are sad.

Significant change in school attendance or decrease in grades is also very common. The youth no longer seems to care about completing homework or worry about grades. He or she may have trouble focusing in class or be found to sleep during class. Many depressed youth begin refusing to go to school due to somatic complaints such as headaches or stomachaches.

DIAGNOSING DEPRESSION

Depression is assessed through a face-to-face clinical interview to determine if an individual meets diagnostic criteria specified by the *Diagnostic and Statistical Manual of Mental Disorders* (*DSM*) for a depressive disorder. In the *DSM*, the three general categories of depression are distinguished by the severity and duration of symptoms. There are very few changes from the *DSM-IV* (4th ed., American Psychiatric Association, 1994) to the *DSM-5* (5th ed., American Psychiatric Association, 2013) for depressive disorders that affect children and adolescents. The most pertinent changes will be addressed within discussions about each type of depression.

Major depression is considered the most serious form of depression. As specified in the *DSM-5*, a person meets the criteria for major depression if he or she has experienced at least five symptoms, one of which is either a depressed mood or a loss of interest or pleasure, during the same two-week period. Other symptoms include significant changes in weight loss or gain (for children this can include failure to reach an expected weight), too much or too little sleep, restlessness or slowed psychomotor functioning, fatigue or loss of energy, feelings of worthlessness or excessive or inappropriate guilt, trouble thinking or concentrating, indecisiveness, and thoughts of death or suicidal ideation (thinking about suicide).

In addition to experiencing at least five of these symptoms, the youth's level of daily functioning must represent a significant decrease from prior functioning. When criteria are met for major depression, the current clinical status or features of the depression are identified with specifiers. The major specifiers for depression in the *DSM-IV* are mild, moderate, severe without psychotic features, and severe with psychotic features. Changes from the *DSM-IV* to *DSM-5* that are of note for diagnosing children or adolescents with major depression are removal of the word *severe* from the specifier *with psychotic symptoms*.

Dysthymia is considered a milder, but more chronic form of depression. The symptoms are not as severe as those of major depression, but they linger for long periods, often two or more years. In order to be diagnosed with dysthymia, a person must experience a depressed mood for most of every day, most days of the week, for at least two years (one year for children). He or she must also experience two or more depressive symptoms, but not have met the criteria for a major depressive episode. Studies have found that somewhere in the range of 10 to 25 percent of persons with dysthymia will go on to develop major depression.

In the *DSM-IV,* depression not otherwise specified (NOS) is a diagnosis given to persons whose depressive symptoms do not meet the criteria for major depression or dysthymia. The difference between receiving a diagnosis of depression NOS rather than major depression is due to not having the specified number (five), level of intensity, or duration of symptoms. Receiving treatment is important regardless of which form of depression a person is experiencing. Without proper treatment, symptoms can continue to worsen. One of the goals for the *DSM-5* workgroups was to eliminate or change NOS as a diagnostic category because it was becoming a catchall for anyone who presented with a disorder, but did not quite meet the criteria. The NOS categories did not include any specific information as to why the diagnosis was made. In the *DSM-5*, NOS has been replaced by not elsewhere classified (American Psychiatric Association, 2013). This diagnosis includes specifiers to explain the clinical condition of a person and why the person did not meet criteria for one of the main depressive disorders.

DEPRESSION IN CHILDREN AND ADOLESCENTS

Depression occurs equally among younger male and female children. However, after puberty, females are twice as likely as males to experience major depression. Once any young person has experienced a depressive episode, he or she is at a high risk of developing another depressive episode. In general, 60 percent of persons who have experienced a major depressive episode will go on to have a second one. A person who experiences major depression as a child is five times more likely to experience major depression as an adult (Cyranowski, Frank, Young, & Shear, 2000; Weissman et al., 1990).

When a young person is assessed for depression, it is important to consider whether the information he or she provides is factual. Some youth may not be open to treatment and therefore may deny having problems. Other youth may lack self-awareness or the ability to communicate their thoughts and feelings, thus making it difficult to determine if there is a problem. It is always important to interview others involved in the youth's life, including a primary caregiver and if possible a teacher or other closely connected persons to get a clear picture of the problems.

SELF-HARMING BEHAVIORS

Self-harm is used as a way to cope with anger, frustration, or emotional pain or to relieve tension. The literature refers to this as non-suicidal self-injury (NSSI). Self-injury refers to a broad range of behaviors, the most common being cutting. Cutting is intentionally scratching or cutting one's body with an object sharp enough to break the skin and make it bleed. People may cut themselves on their legs, belly, arms, or wrists, usually in places where they can hide the injury with clothing. Other self-injuring behaviors (not exhaustive) are listed below:

- Severe pinching with fingernails or other objects to the point of bleeding;
- Banging or punching objects or oneself to the point of bruising or bleeding;
- Biting to the point that bleeding occurs or marks remain on the skin;
- Pulling out hair, eyelashes, or eyebrows;
- Burning the skin;
- Embedding objects into the skin.

Self-injuring behaviors generally take place in private and are hidden by the person, making this phenomenon difficult to research or understand. Research in this area is in its infancy and is primarily based on clinical samples and not the general population. Study results have been mixed. Self-injuring behaviors can start as early as age seven, but most often begin in middle adolescence between the ages of twelve and fifteen. Self-injuring behaviors can last well into adulthood. They can be an indication of depression or another psychiatric illness.

Although the intent of self-harm is not to commit suicide, this behavior may be a sign of suicidal ideation.

Self-injury is strongly linked to childhood abuse, especially sexual abuse. Self-injuring behavior is also linked to eating disorders, substance abuse, post-traumatic stress disorder, borderline personality disorder, depression, and anxiety disorders (Yates, 2004). Teenage girls seem to be at most risk of self-injuring behaviors, but boys often engage in this behavior (Cyranowski et al., 2000). Sexual orientation is also linked to self-injury. Bisexual and questioning youth are at higher risk than their heterosexual peers.

Teenagers cut themselves for various reasons. Most self-injury experts agree that cutting does show some addictive qualities and may serve as a form of self-medication for some individuals. For some people cutting is a way to cope with the pain of strong emotions, intense pressure, or relationship problems. Often individuals who cut do not know how to talk about their feelings; they cut to express strong feelings of rage, sorrow, rejection, desperation, and loneliness.

Individuals who engage in self-injuring behavior often do so to avoid suicide and as a means of relieving pain and/or feeling something. The purpose of self-injury is often the opposite of suicide; the objective is generally to feel better, not to end life. Although 60 percent of individuals with cutting history report not considering suicide, non-suicidal self-injury may best be understood as a symptom of distress that, if it does not relieve the pain, may lead to suicidal behavior (Whitlock & Knox, 2007). It is important to emphasize that individuals with a history of self-injury are at a higher risk for suicide ideation and need to be assessed for suicide risk.

The Centers for Disease Control and Prevention (Eaton et al., 2012) estimates that approximately 14 percent of high school students seriously consider suicide each year, 11 percent have a suicide plan, and 6 percent attempt suicide. Many if not most of these teens never receive mental health services. Major depression is not the only mental health disorder associated with suicidal behavior; other mental health disorders range from eating, anxiety, psychotic, and substance use disorders to behavioral disorders (Shaffer et al., 1996).

Suicide is the third leading cause of death for youth from ages ten to twenty-four, resulting in approximately 149,000 emergency room visits and more than 4,500 deaths in the United States each year (Husky et al., 2012). The U.S. surgeon general estimates that more than 90 percent of children and adolescents who take their lives have a mental health disorder such as depression. Sadly, it has been found that most adolescents who are considering suicide or who have attempted suicide do not get needed mental health treatment (Husky et al., 2012; Luoma, Pearson, & Martin, 2002). Luoma and colleagues suggest that less than half of teens who attempt suicide received mental health services in the year prior to their attempt. Those who did receive mental health treatment appeared to have terminated treatment prematurely. This suggests a need to understand the reasons for early termination and to develop strategies to improve treatment completion.

As addressed in the section on cognitive development in chapter 3, teenagers have the capacity for new thinking during adolescence. They can imagine a perfect world; cognitively they explore solutions to problems and imagine an array of possibilities before them. Although this increase in cognitive sophistication is tremendous, it also opens the door to thinking about various possibilities, including death for some teens. In addition, teens face many stressors. They have access to drugs and alcohol as well as guns, which are readily available in today's society, and they may have fewer social supports than before. With many parents working and time spent alone at home watching TV or playing video games, teens can easily isolate themselves today. Adolescents who are depressed may experience family problems, have emotional problems, and may contemplate suicide. They may exhibit warning signs including changes in sleeping and eating, and they may become agitated easily and neglect their personal appearance. They may see death as one of many options to escape circumstances they consider unbearable. Suicidal ideation becomes a major threat when the person (1) has a plan for death, (2) has the means to accomplish the plan, and (3) lacks supervision so that time for actualizing the plan is available.

Suicidal ideation in teens should always be taken seriously and assessed properly. There are two types of teens who generally commit suicide. The first type includes intelligent and withdrawn teens who fail to meet their own standards, and the second is teens with delinquent and antisocial behavior (Lehnert, Overholser, & Spirito, 1994).

Risk and Protective Factors

Risk factors are characteristics associated with suicide. They are not necessarily the direct cause of suicide, but they are contributors to the increased risk for suicide. Protective factors are characteristics that buffer against suicide. When suicidal ideation is assessed, these factors should be considered. For instance, a higher risk of suicide exists for youth who have previously attempted suicide or have a family member who committed suicide. Drug and alcohol use or abuse increases the risk of suicide. Gender and race/ethnicity are factors. Males are more likely to die from a suicide attempt than females (83% compared to 17%). Hispanic and Native American/Alaskan Native youth have higher rates of suicide than white non-Hispanic or black youth. According to the Centers for Disease Control and Prevention (Eaton et al., 2012), risk and protective factors associated with suicide include those listed in Table 4.1.

Warning Signs

Most often (4 out of 5 times), suicidal teens exhibit clear warning signs. Clear warning signs include an obsession with death that is evidenced through a

Table 4.1. Risk and protective factors associated with suicide

Risk factors
- Family history of suicide;
- Family history of child maltreatment;
- Previous suicide attempt(s);
- History of mental disorders, particularly clinical depression;
- History of alcohol and substance abuse;
- Feelings of hopelessness;
- Impulsive or aggressive tendencies;
- Cultural and religious beliefs about suicide (e.g., belief that suicide is a noble resolution of a personal dilemma);
- Local epidemics of suicide;
- Isolation, or a feeling of being cut off from other people;
- Barriers to accessing mental health treatment;
- Loss (relational, social, work, or financial);
- Physical illness;
- Easy access to lethal methods;
- Unwillingness to seek help.

Protective factors
- Effective clinical care for mental, physical, and substance abuse disorders;
- Easy access to a variety of clinical interventions and support for help seeking;
- Family and community support (connectedness);
- Support from ongoing medical and mental health care relationships;
- Skills in problem solving, conflict resolution, and nonviolent ways of handling disputes;
- Cultural and religious beliefs that discourage suicide and support instincts for self-preservation.

youth's conversations, writings, music, or artwork. Youth may stop participating in things they once enjoyed. Often suicidal youth will experience extreme changes in their personality and behaviors, including irrational or bizarre behavior. Making direct or indirect suicidal threats and giving away belongings are also common. The U.S. Department of Health and Human Services offers the mnemonic *IS PATH WARM?* as a tool to identify red flags indicating suicidal ideation:

- Ideation—threatened or communicated
- Substance abuse—excessive or increased
- Purposeless—no reasons for living
- Anxiety—agitation/insomnia
- Trapped—feeling there is no way out
- Hopelessness
- Withdrawing—from friends, family, society
- Anger (uncontrolled)—rage, seeking revenge
- Recklessness—risky acts, unthinking
- Mood changes (dramatic)

Addressing Suicidal Ideation

Too often, warning signs go ignored because we believe that the person is just trying to get attention. It is common for people to refuse to believe that a young person would follow through with taking his or her own life. There is also a mistaken belief that a discussion of suicide may increase someone's suicidal ideation. Both of these are myths. Young people do commit suicide, and discussing and questioning a youth about suicidal ideation will not put the idea of suicide into his or her head or result in increased suicidality. Ignoring the warning signs can result in serious consequences.

If you identify or suspect suicidal ideation, it is important to address the issue head on. Question the youth as to whether he or she is having thoughts about harming himself or herself. If you find that the young person is having suicidal ideation, determine if he or she has a determined time frame and a plan for committing suicide. A youth with imminent suicidal ideation, meaning that he or she has a plan and the means to carry it out, should never be left alone. It is important that he or she gets connected to a mental health professional and that someone, usually the primary caregiver, knows about the situation and promises to watch the youth and ensure that he or she gets professional care. If the threat or attempt of suicide is serious, psychiatric hospitalization may be indicated as a means of monitoring the youth to ensure safety and offer intensive treatment.

Suicide contracts are a controversial preventative intervention that many counselors, therapists, and sometimes even family members try to implement. In such a contract, the suicidal person is asked to sign a document agreeing not to harm himself or herself. The document, which is not a legal document, sets out a plan and a promise to call someone rather than hurting himself or herself. The controversy with this intervention is that a person may appear to agree with the contract and sign it, but then not follow through with the agreement. There is also a phenomenon known as *flight into health*. Sometimes people with suicidal intent will suddenly say that they feel better and no longer plan to commit suicide as a way to be left alone so that they can kill themselves. It is important to assess whether the youth is presenting with a sudden flight into health rather than an actual decrease in suicidal ideation.

SCREENING TOOLS

There are many valid and reliable rating scales that can be used to screen children for depression. Many of these tools can be administered by a pediatrician, the school social worker, child welfare workers, counselors, or other professionals working with children. Some of these tools are available free. Others are subject to copyright and require permission for use or purchase. Following are a few examples of measurement tools for assessing depression.

Children's Depression Rating Scale-Revised

The Children's Depression Rating Scale-Revised (CDRS-R), developed by Poznanski and Mokros (1996), was designed for assessing depressive symptoms in six- to twelve-year-olds. It is also a useful tool for measuring response to treatment across time. The CDRS-R is administered through a semi-structured interview conducted with either the youth or an adult who knows the child well. It takes approximately fifteen to twenty minutes to administer. It was designed to rate across seventeen symptom areas, including the *DSM* criteria for depression. The CDRS-R can be purchased online from Western Psychological Services.

Center for Epidemiological Studies Depression Scale Modified for Children

The Center for Epidemiological Studies Depression Scale Modified for Children (CES-DC) is a self-report tool designed for assessing depression in youth from ages six to seventeen (Faulstich, Carey, Ruggiero, Enyart, & Gresham, 1986; Radloff, 1977). The CES-DC is a self-administered twenty-item scale. Youth are asked to rate the level to which they have experienced certain feelings. This scale takes about five minutes to complete and can be downloaded free from Bright Futures (http://www.brightfutures.org).

The Beck Depression Inventory for Youth and the Beck Depression Inventory-II Student

The Beck Depression Inventory for Youth (BDI-Y) for ages seven to fourteen and the Beck Depression Inventory-II (BDI-II) Student for ages thirteen and older are commonly used tools for early identification and screening of depressive symptoms (Beck, Ward, & Mendelson, 1961). The BDI-Y consists of twenty self-report items that are written at a second grade level. The BDI-II consists of twenty-one self-report items. Both tools take between five and ten minutes to complete and can be purchased from Pearson (http://www.pearsonclinical.com).

CASE STUDIES

Following are case studies that relate to depression. In the next chapter, we will explore evidence-based treatments and practices for depression. We will return to the case studies presented here to learn about the actual types of interventions that were provided to the youth in the studies and to learn to determine which intervention is the most appropriate.

Mary

Mary is a sixteen-year-old in the ninth grade. Her family is considered a very loving upper class family. Mary made straight A's and rarely missed a day of school through elementary and middle school. She took piano lessons and played the trumpet in the school band. She was very involved in the youth group at her church. About midway through the ninth grade, Mary started complaining of stomachaches and refused to go to school. She did this two to three times a week. When she stayed at home, she stayed in bed and slept. She ate very little at meals. Mary's mother took her to see her primary care physician. Her doctor ran all sorts of medical tests to determine the cause of her stomach problems. No medical cause could be found. Mary continued to complain and missed school. She got to the point where she refused to go to school altogether. She did not pick up her trumpet, play her piano, or hang out with her church youth group. She missed so much school that her grades went from A's to F's and she was at risk of having to repeat the ninth grade.

Following are some questions about Mary's case:

1.   What symptoms was Mary experiencing?

2.   Does she meet the criteria for a diagnosis of any of the types of depression? Explain. If she does, which one?

3.   Based on your current knowledge, what interventions would you suggest? Do you believe that the appropriate intervention or treatment was provided?

4.   Who should be included in the treatment planning and interventions?

5.   What barriers might get in the way of effectively intervening?

6.   What suggestions/thoughts/ideas do you have for the other members of her family?

David

David was nine years old when his father died. After the death of his father, David's behavior changed. He started to exhibit aggressive behavior. He tormented and hit his younger brother for no obvious reason. He began to sit in his tree house by himself for hours on end drawing bloody and gruesome pictures of monsters killing people. In school, he had difficulty focusing on and completing his work. When his teacher tried to redirect him, he started yelling that he sucked and could not do the assignment because he was stupid. Sometimes when he was asked to do the simplest of tasks at home, he would bang his head on the floor or hit walls. After approximately six weeks of this new behavior, his mother decided to take him to see a mental health professional.

Consider the following questions:

1. What symptoms was David experiencing?
2. Does he meet the criteria for a diagnosis of any of the types of depression? Explain. If he does, which one?
3. Based on your current knowledge, what interventions would you suggest? Do you believe that the appropriate intervention or treatment was provided?
4. Who should be included in the treatment planning and interventions?
5. What barriers might get in the way of effectively intervening?
6. What suggestions/thoughts/ideas do you have for the other members of his family?

REFERENCES

American Psychiatric Association. (1994). *Diagnostic and statistical manual of mental disorders* (4th ed.). Washington, DC: Author.

American Psychiatric Association. (2013). *Diagnostic and statistical manual of mental disorders* (5th ed.). Washington, DC: Author.

Beck, A. T., Ward, C., & Mendelson, M. (1961). Beck depression inventory (BDI). *Archives of General Psychiatry, 4*, 561–571.

Cyranowski, J. M., Frank, E., Young, E., & Shear, M. K. (2000). Adolescent onset of the gender difference in lifetime rates of major depression. *Archives of General Psychiatry, 57*, 21–27.

Eaton, D. K., Kann, L., Kinchen, S., Shanklin, S., Flint, K. H., Hawkins, J., . . . Wechsler, H. (2012). Youth risk behavior surveillance—United States, 2011. *Morbidity and Mortality Weekly Report, 61*(4). Retrieved from http://www.cdc.gov/mmwr/pdf/ss/ss 6104.pdf

Faulstich, M. E., Carey, M. P., Ruggiero, L., Enyart, P., & Gresham, F. (1986). Assessment of depression in childhood and adolescence. An evaluation of the Center for Epidemiological Studies Depression Scale for Children (CES-DC). *American Journal of Psychiatry, 143*, 1024–1027.

Husky, M., Olfson, M., He, J., Nock, M., Swanson, S., & Merikangas, K. (2012). Twelve-month suicidal symptoms and use of services among adolescents: Results from the National Comorbidity Survey. *Psychiatric Services, 63*, 989–996.

Kandel, E. R., Schwartz, J. H., & Jessell, T. M. (2000). *Principles of neural science* (4th ed.). New York: McGraw-Hill.

Krishnan, K., Taylor, W. D., McQuoid, D. R., MacFall, J. R., Payne, M. E., Provenzale, J. M., & Steffens, D. C. (2004). Clinical characteristics of magnetic resonance imaging-defined subcortical ischemic depression. *Biological Psychiatry, 55,* 390–397.

Lehnert, K., Overholser, J., & Spirito, A. (1994). Internalized and externalized anger in adolescent suicide attempters. *Journal of Adolescent Research, 9,* 105–119.

Luoma, J. B., Pearson, J. L., & Martin, C. E. (2002). Contact with mental health and primary care prior to suicide: A review of the evidence. *American Journal of Psychiatry, 159,* 909–916.

Merikangas, K. R., He, J., Burstein, M., Swanson, S. A., Avenevoli, S., Cui, L., . . . Swendsen, J. (2010). Lifetime prevalence of mental disorders in U.S. adolescents: Results from the National Comorbidity Study-Adolescent Supplement (NCS-A). *Journal of the American Academy of Child & Adolescent Psychiatry, 49,* 980–989.

National Institute of Mental Health. (n.d.-a). *Depression in children and adolescents.* Retrieved from http://www.nimh.nih.gov/health/topics/depression/depression-in -children-and-adolescents.shtml

National Institute of Mental Health. (n.d.-b). *Suicide: A major, preventable mental health problem: Facts about suicide and suicide prevention among teens and young adults.* Retrieved from http://www.nimh.nih.gov/health/publications/suicide-a-major-pre ventable-mental-health-problem-fact-sheet/teen-suicide.pdf

Poznanski, M. D., & Mokros, H. B. (1996). *Children's depression rating scale-Revised* (CDRS-R). Los Angeles: Western Psychological Services.

Radloff, L. S. (1977). The CES-D scale: A self-report depression scale for research in the general population. *Applied Psychological Measurement, 1,* 385–401.

Shaffer, D., Gould, M. S., Fisher, P., Trautman, P., Moreau, D., Kleinman, M., & Flory, M. (1996). Psychiatric diagnosis in child and adolescent suicide. *Archives of General Psychiatry, 53,* 339–348.

Tsuang, M. T., & Faraone, S. V. (1990). *The genetics of mood disorders.* Baltimore, MD: Johns Hopkins University Press.

Weissman, M. M., Wolk, S., Goldstein, R. B., Moreau, D., Adams, P., Greenwald, S., . . . Wichramaratne, P. (1990). Depressed adolescents grown up. *Journal of the American Medical Association, 281,* 1701–1713.

Whitlock, J. L., & Knox, K. (2007). The relationship between suicide and self-injury in a young adult population. *Archives of Pediatrics and Adolescent Medicine, 161,* 634–640. Retrieved from http://www.selfinjury.bctr.cornell.edu/publications/a3.pdf

Yates, T. M. (2004). The developmental psychopathology of self-injurious behavior: Compensatory regulation in posttraumatic adaptation. *Clinical Psychological Review, 24,* 35–74.

CHAPTER 5

Treatment of Depressive Disorders

MEDICATION AND PSYCHOTHERAPY are the two most common treatments for depression. Eighty percent of persons who receive treatment experience improvement in their depression (National Institute of Mental Health, 2005). The type of treatment prescribed by a doctor depends on the type and level of depression. Medication is indicated mostly for persons with major depression, although it can be used to treat less severe forms of depression as well. Medication does not provide a cure, but it can help the body regulate its own chemistry to control the symptoms of depression. The amount of control varies from person to person. Psychotherapy helps a person change faulty thinking and poor coping into positive thinking and coping. Research has found that a combination of medication and psychotherapy has the best results in reducing levels of depression.

ANTIDEPRESSANT MEDICATION

There are currently approximately twenty-five different antidepressant medications that help the body regulate the neurotransmitters dopamine, serotonin, and/ or norepinephrine in the brain. These neurotransmitters are essential for normal brain activity. There are four main classes of antidepressants, each acting on different neurotransmitters: serotonin reuptake inhibitors, serotonin norepinephrine reuptake inhibitors, monoamine oxidase inhibitors, and tricyclic antidepressants. Different people will respond to these medications differently (Trivedi et al., 2006). It is not easy to determine in advance which medication a person will respond to best.

The most popularly prescribed antidepressants are Prozac, Paxil, Lexapro, Celexa, and Zoloft. These medications are in the class of selective serotonin reuptake inhibitors (SSRIs), meaning that they affect the concentration and activity of one specific neurotransmitter in the brain known as serotonin. The SSRIs are popular due to their high level of effectiveness in reducing symptoms and due to their low risk of side effects and overdoses. This class of medication is the most popular for treating children and adolescents. Table 5.1 lists selective SSRI medications by brand and generic names.

A newer class of medications is the serotonin norepinephrine reuptake inhibitors (SNRIs). This class of medications has been found to be effective in alleviating symptoms of depression and anxiety. The SNRIs target both the serotonin and the norepinephrine in the brain. As shown in Table 5.2, examples of SNRI medications include Pristiq, Cymbalta, and Effexor. The SSRIs and SNRIs have been found to have relatively equal response rates.

Table 5.1. Selective serotonin reuptake inhibitors

Brand name	Generic name
Celexa	Citalopram
Lexapro	Escitalopram
Luvox	Fluvoxamine
Luvox CR	Paroxetine
Paxil	Fluoxetine
Prozac	Sertraline
Zoloft	

Table 5.2. Serotonin norepinephrine reuptake inhibitors

Brand name	Generic name
Cymbalta	Duloxetine
Effexor XR	Venlafaxine
Pristiq	Desvenlafaxine

There are atypical antidepressants that have been approved by the U.S. Food and Drug Administration (FDA) for treating depression. Each of these medications works differently from other atypical antidepressants and from the other classes of antidepressants. What they have in common with each other and with other antidepressants is that they affect dopamine, serotonin, and/or norepinephrine in some way that changes the balance of these neurotransmitters to affect mood. The exact way in which they affect the neurotransmitters is unknown. These medications share common side effects: dry mouth, constipation, and dizziness. In addition, each one causes side effects that are different from those caused by the others. Table 5.3 lists atypical medications.

Tricyclic antidepressants (TCAs) and monoamine oxidase inhibitors (MAOIs) are older classes of antidepressants. Both tricyclics and MAOIs are far less expensive than the other two classes of medications and come in generic forms; however, there is a high risk of side effects. Tricyclics affect serotonin and norephinephrine, and MAOIs block the effect of an enzyme in the brain that prevents the breakdown of serotonin and norephinephrine. Tricyclic overdose is a serious issue because it does not take much more than a normal dosage to cause an overdose. Overdose is also a serious issue for MAOIs. In addition to the long list of side effects of MAOIs, there is a risk of experiencing a severe spike in blood pressure. Although these medications are not the first line of antidepressants prescribed, they are still prescribed to people who do not respond to the

Table 5.3. Atypical medications

Brand name	Generic name
Wellbutrin	Bupropion
Remeron	Mirtazapine
Nefazodone (discontinued)	Dutonin, Nefadar, Serzone
Oleptro	Trazodone

newer medications. Brand names and generic names of tricyclic antidepressants and monoamine oxidase inhibitors are listed in Tables 5.4 and 5.5, respectively.

ANTIDEPRESSANT MEDICATION USE IN CHILDREN AND ADOLESCENTS

Unfortunately, few of the antidepressants have been studied in children or adolescents. Prozac is currently the only antidepressant approved for treating children under the age of eight. However, antidepressants are commonly prescribed and can be effective for children. When a medication has not been studied and approved by the FDA to treat certain conditions or certain ages, it is prescribed *off label*. Although SSRI antidepressants are the most frequently prescribed for young people, research studies have found a link between SSRI and SNRI medications and increased suicidal thoughts and behaviors. A review of data from twenty-four clinical trials evaluating the effectiveness of antidepressants on children and adolescents revealed an increased risk for suicidality in the youths taking antidepressants compared to the control group who received a placebo

Table 5.4. Tricyclic antidepressants

Brand name	Generic name
Adapin	Doxepin
Anafranil	Clomiprimine
Aventyl	Nortriptyline
Elavil	Amitriptyline
Ludiomil	Maprotiline
Norpramin	Desipramine
Pamelor	Nortriptyline
Sinequan	Doxepin
Surmontil	Trimipramine
Tofranil	Imipramine
Vivactil	Protriptyline

Table 5.5. Monoamine oxidase inhibitors

Brand name	Generic name
Marplan	Isocarboxid Phenelzine
Nardil	Tranylcypromine
Parnate	

(Bridge et al., 2007). Due to the findings of this review, the FDA gave SSRI and SNRI medications black box warnings, the most serious medication warning given by the FDA. These warnings appear on the labels of prescription medications to alert consumers of any serious safety concerns (i.e., serious side effects or life-threatening risks). The classes of SSRI and SNRI medications have been given this warning due to the increased risk of suicide they can cause in young people.

When a youth is prescribed an antidepressant, it is important to monitor him or her for unusual changes in behavior and suicidal ideation. When prescribing an antidepressant, the doctor must weigh the increased risk of suicide against the potential benefit of the medication. Untreated persons who are depressed are at an increased risk of attempting or committing suicide as well.

COGNITIVE-BEHAVIORAL THERAPY

Cognitive-behavioral therapy (CBT) is the most extensively tested psychosocial treatment for depression. It has been found to be effective in treating both children and adolescents experiencing depression (Burns & Hoagwood, 2002; Burns, Hoagwood, & Mrazek, 1999; Jensen, Weersing, Hoagwood, & Goldman, 2005; Kazdin & Weisz, 1998). Developed in the 1960s by Aaron T. Beck, CBT focuses on changing how one thinks and acts as a means of improving depression. This is based on the theory that depression is both caused and maintained by negative or irrational beliefs that affect behavior (Beck, 1967, 1970; Clark, Beck, & Alford, 1999). When people learn to recognize and evaluate the rationality of these negative, irrational beliefs, they can replace them with healthier thoughts and change their negative behaviors to healthier ones. This in effect will improve their mood. Because CBT has been extensively tested and found effective in treating depression, it is often a cornerstone in evidence-based treatments for depression.

Cognitive-behavioral therapy is structured and time limited, lasting from fourteen to sixteen weeks. Treatment is goal oriented and focuses on the what and how of specific problems occurring in the immediate present. Cognitive-behavioral therapy does not focus on the why of a person's thinking. The first goal of CBT is to help youth realize that they can control their own behaviors and therefore can change their depression. This technique is known as *cognitive restructuring*. The therapist works with the youth to change irrational and negative thought patterns by teaching strategies to stop, confront, and change these thought patterns.

The client takes an active role in treatment. Mood diaries or emotions charts are common tools used to assist the young person to monitor thoughts, actions, physiological sensations, emotions, and events and to become aware of how these factors affect depression. The therapist also teaches the youth problem-solving, coping, self-monitoring, relaxation, and social skills. Learning ways to relax in stressful situations helps the youth feel more competent and opens the door to trying out other skills. Homework is used as a strategy for increasing learning and integrating the skills being developed.

Penn Resiliency Program

The Penn Resiliency Program (PRP) is a curriculum-based intervention aimed at promoting resilience and prevention of depressive symptoms in youth from ages ten to fourteen. It was developed by Karen Reivich and Jane Gillham at the University of Pennsylvania. This program has been highly researched and found to be effective in youth across ethnic and culturally diverse populations (Brunwasser, Gillham, & Kim, 2009; Cardemil, Reivich, Beevers, Seligman, & James, 2007). It uses a small group format that can be applied in schools or in clinical settings. The curriculum can be used by teachers, counselors, or therapists.

The first five sessions of PRP utilize cognitive-behavioral techniques aimed at helping youth identify their self-talk and faulty thinking and learn to adapt their thinking to be more flexible. Youth learn about the link between thoughts and feelings and different thinking styles, thereby challenging their thinking. The remainder of the sessions (6–12) focus on teaching the youth coping, problem-solving, assertiveness and negotiating, decision-making, and social skills aimed at helping them manage day-to-day stressors. In all of the sessions, youth practice their new skills through games and activities. More information on PRP can be found at http://www.ppc.sas.upenn.edu/prpsum.htm.

Adolescents Coping with Depression

Adolescents Coping with Depression (CWD-A) was designed for adolescents from ages twelve to eighteen (Lewinsohn, Clarke, Hops, & Andrews,

1990). It is a cognitive-behavioral intervention conducted in small groups of four to ten youths. The curriculum consists of sixteen 2-hour sessions. The focus of CWD-A is on helping youth monitor their mood, change unrealistic thinking, increase participation in pleasant activities, and decrease anxiety. As with the other interventions using a CBT approach, adolescents are taught new skills such as social skills, communication skills, and conflict resolution. The manual for CWD-A is accompanied by a workbook for group participants. The workbook includes parallel exercises for each session as well as homework exercises.

Adolescents Coping with Depression also includes materials for a caregiver group to accompany the youth group. The caregiver group focuses on teaching caregivers about adolescent depression and describing the skills being taught to the youth. In addition, caregivers are taught how to better communicate with and support children as they work through their depression. Caregivers also have a workbook and complete homework assignments. For more information, visit http://www.kpchr.org/research/public/acwd/acwd.html.

Interpersonal Psychotherapy

Interpersonal psychotherapy (IPT) was originally developed to treat adults experiencing depression (Mufson, Pollack Dora, Moreau, & Weissman, 2004). It has since been found to be effective in treating adolescents experiencing depression. It is a very didactic therapy with overarching goals to decrease depressive symptoms and improve interpersonal relationships. The underlying basis of IPT is that depression can be caused, maintained, or buffered by the quality of relationships with others.

Interpersonal Psychotherapy for Depressed Adolescents

Interpersonal Psychotherapy for Depressed Adolescents (IPT-A) is a manualized version of IPT (Mufson et al., 1994). The treatment consists of twelve to sixteen individual sessions. This program was developed to address relationship problems specific to adolescence such as interpersonal relationships with the opposite sex, problems with parental authority, and peer pressure. It is meant to be implemented by master's or doctoral level clinicians.

The first focus of IPT is to provide education on the causes, correlates, and etiology of depression; to explore the youth's interpersonal relationships with others; and to identify a specific problem area that will be targeted during treatment. Once the problem area has been identified, the therapist educates the youth on the connection between relationship problems and depression. The next strategy of IPT is to help the youth clarify expectations of relationships and teach them new skills aimed at improving significant relationships. During sessions, the youth practices the new skills with the therapist through role playing. Once a certain level of mastery is achieved, the youth uses the techniques outside of therapy sessions. Through this process, the therapist helps link improvement in mood to the new ways of communicating with others. More information is available at http://interpersonalpsychotherapy.org/ipt-for-adolescents.

CASE STUDIES

Mary

Mary is the sixteen-year-old from a loving upper class family. She did very well in school, making straight A's and having near perfect attendance through elementary and middle school. She was actively involved in many extracurricular activities.

About midway through the ninth grade, Mary began having somatic complaints and missed two to three days of school each week. She slept more than usual and ate much less than usual. She went from being a straight A student to being an F student. No medical cause could be found for these changes. Her primary care doctor suggested that she see a counselor.

Her mother spoke with friends to find a counselor. She was referred to a counselor who was trained in CBT. Mary's mood improved some after three weeks of counseling, but she was still experiencing depressive symptoms. Her counselor referred Mary to a psychiatrist. The psychiatrist started Mary on a low dose of Paxil. After two weeks on the medication, her mood improved significantly. She continued with counseling for the full twelve sessions of CBT.

Each week while she was on the medication and receiving counseling, Mary continued to improve. By the end of CBT, she was feeling like her old self. Her mother set an appointment for Mary and her to meet with the school counselor and all Mary's teachers. As a group, they came up with a plan to help Mary get her grades up. She was allowed to retake tests that she had failed and redo major assignments. She was able to complete these things while keeping up with her other school work.

David

David is the nine-year-old whose father had passed away. After the death of his father, his behavior changed drastically. He became very aggressive toward others. He began to isolate himself and to draw death-themed pictures. At school, he had difficulty focusing on and completing his work. When asked to do the simplest of tasks at home or school, he would bang his head on the floor or hit walls. After approximately six weeks of this behavior, his mother took him to see a therapist.

The therapist helped David talk about the loss of his father. She worked with him to express his feelings, either verbally or through art. She taught him relaxation techniques to use when he felt stressed. David maintained a diary, in which he wrote down the activities of his day and his feelings about the activities. The therapist used the diary to help David change his negative thoughts into active coping strategies.

For the last fifteen minutes of each session, David's mother joined in the session. The therapist modeled and taught her how to respond in supportive ways to David's emotions. After eight sessions, David was expressing his feelings better and experiencing a significant decrease in aggressive behavior.

Study Questions

1. What do these real life scenarios have in common?

2. What are the differences?

3. After you learned what happened to each of the youths, do you have any different thoughts on how you would have handled the situation if you were the families' social worker?

REFERENCES

Beck, A. T. (1967). *The diagnosis and management of depression.* Philadelphia: University of Pennsylvania Press.

Beck, A. T. (1970). *Depression: Causes and treatment.* Philadelphia: University of Pennsylvania Press.

Bridge, J. A., Iyengar, S., Salary, C. B., Barbe, R. P., Birmaher, B., Pincus, H. A., . . . Brent, D. A. (2007). Clinical response and risk for reported suicidal ideation and suicide attempts in pediatric antidepressant treatment, a meta-analysis of randomized controlled trials. *Journal of the American Medical Association, 297*, 1683–1696.

Brunwasser, S. M., Gillham, J. E., & Kim, E. S. (2009). A meta-analytic review of the Penn Resiliency Program's effect on depressive symptoms. *Journal of Consulting and Clinical Psychology, 77*, 1042–1054.

Burns, B. J., & Hoagwood, K. (Eds.). (2002). *Community treatment for youth: Evidence-based interventions for severe emotional and behavioral disorders.* New York: Oxford University Press.

Burns, B. J., Hoagwood, K., & Mrazek, P. J. (1999). Effective treatment for mental disorders in children and adolescents. *Clinical Child and Family Psychology Review, 2*, 199–254.

Cardemil, E. V., Reivich, K. J., Beevers, C. G., Seligman, M. E. P., & James, J. (2007). The prevention of depressive symptoms in low-income, minority children: Two-year follow-up. *Behaviour Research and Therapy, 45*, 313–327.

Clark, D. A., Beck, A. T., & Alford, B. A. (1999). *Scientific foundations of cognitive theory and therapy of depression.* New York: John Wiley.

Jensen, P. S., Weersing, R., Hoagwood, K. E., & Goldman, E. (2005). What is the evidence for evidence-based treatments? A hard look at our soft underbelly. *Mental Health Services Research, 7*, 53–74.

Kazdin, A. E., & Weisz, J. R. (1998). Identifying and developing empirically supported child and adolescent treatments. *Journal of Counseling and Clinical Psychology, 66*, 19–36.

Lewinsohn, P. M., Clarke, G. N., Hops, H., & Andrews, J. (1990). Cognitive-behavioral group treatment of depression in adolescents. *Behavior Therapy, 21*, 385–401.

Mufson, L., Moreau, D., Weissman, M. M., Wickramaratne, P., Martin, J., & Samoilov, A. (1994). Modification of interpersonal psychotherapy with depressed adolescents (IPT-A): Phase I and phase II studies. *Journal of the American Academy of Child and Adolescent Psychiatry, 33*, 695–705.

Mufson, L., Pollack Dorta, K., Moreau, D., & Weissman, M. (2004). *Interpersonal psychotherapy for depressed adolescents.* New York: Guilford Press.

National Institute of Mental Health. (2005). *Antidepressant medications for children and adolescents: Information for parents and caregivers.* Retrieved from http://www .nimh.nih.gov/about/updates/2005/antidepressant-medications-for-children-and -adolescents-information-for-parents-and-caregivers.shtml

Trivedi, M. H., Fava, M., Wisniewski, S. R., Thase, M. E., Quitkin, F., Warden, D., . . . Rush, J. A. (2006). Medication augmentation after the failure of SSRIs for depression. *New England Journal of Medicine, 354*, 1243–1252.

CHAPTER 6

Anxiety Disorders

OF ALL THE MENTAL HEALTH PROBLEMS experienced by children and adolescents, anxiety disorders are the most common. Anxiety, stress, and worry are normal feelings until they severely interfere with daily life. Anxiety disorders include disorders that share features of excessive stress, anxiety, and fear. The anxiety experienced is the anticipation that something unpleasant is going to happen, and in response, a person experiences physical and biological reactions that are not due to a medical problem (American Psychiatric Association, 2013). The responses may include an increase in heart rate, profuse sweating, heartburn, headaches or other body aches, gastrointestinal problems, or nausea, for example. Anxiety disorders include posttraumatic stress disorder, generalized anxiety disorder, social phobia, panic disorder, and specific phobias. Obsessive-compulsive disorder was moved from the anxiety disorders section in the *DSM-IV* (American Psychiatric Association, 1994) to the section "Obsessive-Compulsive and Related Disorders" in the *DSM-5* (American Psychiatric Association, 2013). Because it shares many similarities with anxiety disorders, it is included in this chapter.

Each anxiety disorder has distinct characteristics, but the symptoms overlap those of other anxiety disorders. An estimated 10 percent of children experience a diagnosable anxiety disorder at some point in their childhood. It is normal for all youth to experience anxiety at different points in their lives. Normal levels of anxiety will usually extinguish when the situation causing the anxiety is resolved or as the youth is able to use coping skills to manage the anxiety. However, when anxiety reaches a level at which it is interrupting daily life for an extended period of time, intervention is needed. Along with anxiety disorders, children or adolescents may experience panic attacks or agoraphobia. Both panic attacks and agoraphobia can occur as part of almost any anxiety disorder, although not all persons with an anxiety disorder experience them.

PANIC ATTACK

Although the *DSM* includes panic disorder, which refers to a disorder in which a person experiences recurrent, unexpected attacks of intense fear or discomfort during times when there is no real danger or threat, panic attacks often occur with other mental health disorders. When this is the case, the panic attack is coded as a *specifier* to the other disorder. The symptoms experienced during a panic attack are very intense and scary for the person experiencing them. They can also be scary for an observer. During a panic attack, a person may feel as if he or she is going crazy or may die. The symptoms of panic attacks are much more intense than the symptoms experienced due strictly to anxiety and can occur in the context of any anxiety disorder and sometimes in conjunction with other disorders. Panic attacks last for a discrete period of time, with the symptoms of the panic peaking within ten minutes. According to the *DSM*, during a true panic attack, four or more of the following symptoms will be experienced:

- Palpitations, pounding heartbeats, or accelerated heart rate;
- Sweating, trembling, or shaking;
- Sensations of shortness of breath or smothering;
- Feelings of choking, chest pain, or discomfort;

- Nausea or abdominal distress;
- Dizziness, unsteadiness, lightheadedness, or faintness;
- Feelings of being outside of reality (called derealization) or detached from oneself (called depersonalization);
- Fear of losing control or going crazy;
- Fear of dying;
- Feelings of numbness or tingling sensations (called paresthesias);
- Chills or hot flushes.

Agoraphobia

Agoraphobia is characterized by extreme fear of being in a place or a situation from which there is no escape, for example, in a large crowd, on a train, or in an elevator. The person may be fearful of losing control in public or experiencing a panic attack in front of others and being embarrassed or not having the help he or she needs. Persons with agoraphobia begin avoiding places or situations in which they feel unsafe or unable to maintain control. As time goes on, they find fewer places where they can go without the fear. Many become prisoners in their own homes.

Panic Disorder with or without Agoraphobia

When a person experiences recurrent, unexpected panic attacks that are not associated with any specific trigger and cannot be attributed to another mental health disorder, substance abuse, or general medical condition, he or she may meet the criteria for panic disorder. For at least one month following an unexpected panic attack, the person must experience ongoing fear of having another attack, excessive worry about the causes or consequences of attacks, and/or a significant change in behavior resulting from the attacks. Panic disorder usually begins during late adolescence or early adulthood. It can begin in childhood, although this is rare. A child or teenager who has a biological parent, sibling, or other first degree relative with a panic disorder is up to eight times more likely to develop a panic disorder (American Psychiatric Association, 2013).

SEPARATION ANXIETY DISORDER

Separation anxiety disorder usually begins in childhood. All children experience separation anxiety as part of normal childhood development beginning around seven months and subsiding by three years of age (American Psychiatric Association, 2013). Approximately 4 to 5 percent of children and 1 to 2 percent of adolescents experience separation anxiety disorder. With this disorder, children and adolescents experience extreme levels of fear and anxiety that are out of proportion to the situation and to their developmental age. This fear and anxiety significantly affect daily functioning and can prevent youth from participating in independent activities, particularly those away from home. They may refuse to go to school or to play with friends for fear of being separated from their family. Older youth may experience excessive worry that something bad will happen to them or their family such as a serious car wreck or the sudden death of a parent.

Diagnosing Separation Anxiety

In order for a youth to be diagnosed with separation anxiety, he or she must be experiencing a level of anxiety that is inappropriate for his or her developmental stage and excessive when he or she is threatened with being separated from home or from an individual with whom he or she is attached, usually a parent. The anxiety must be so severe that it significantly interferes with daily functioning or relationships. According to the *DSM-5*, to be diagnosed with separation anxiety, the youth must exhibit three or more of the following symptoms over a time span of at least four weeks:

- Recurrent excessive distress when separation from home or major attachment figures occurs or is anticipated
- Persistent and excessive worry about losing or having harm befall major attachment figures
- Persistent and excessive worry that an untoward event will lead to separation from a major attachment figure (e.g., getting lost or kidnapped)
- Reluctance or refusal to go to school or elsewhere because of fear of separation
- Persistent and excessive fear of or reluctance to be alone or without major attachment figures at home or without significant adults in other settings
- Persistent reluctance or refusal to go to sleep without being near a major attachment figure or to sleep away from home

- Repeated nightmares involving the theme of separation
- Repeated complaints of physical symptoms (such as headaches, stomachaches, nausea, or vomiting) when separation from major attachment figures occurs or is anticipated

SOCIAL PHOBIA

Social phobia is considered one of the most common mental health disorders, affecting nearly 13 percent of people across their lifespan. Someone who experiences social phobia has excessive fear about being in certain social situations. We all experience some level of nervousness in situations in which we have to give a speech or presentation or perform in front of others. Although we are nervous, we are able to give the speech or perform. People with social phobia experience extreme fear of and anxiety about being judged or evaluated by other people. The fear experienced is unreasonable for the situation and severely interferes with a person's functioning. A person who is exposed to the feared situation experiences severe anxiety symptoms such as a panic attack.

Persons with social phobia are often characterized as being quiet, shy, aloof, nervous, or unfriendly. Their fear can interfere with their ability to be social or make friends. It is not the case that they do not want to be part of a social group or develop friendships; it is the extreme fear that paralyzes them and prevents them from engaging in such interactions.

Diagnosing Social Phobia

To be diagnosed with social phobia, a person must meet the criteria specified in the *DSM*. First is a persistent fear of social situations in which a person perceives that others may scrutinize him or her, or in which he or she may act in a way that is embarrassing or humiliating. The fear of these social situations results in significant levels of anxiety. The person either avoids these situations or endures them with intense anxiety or distress. Secondly, adults must recognize that their anxiety is excessive or out of proportion for the situation. The response to the anxiety may take the form of a panic attack or other extreme responses. The level of anxiety or distress must interfere with daily living. The symptoms must not be attributable to a medical condition or another mental health problem.

Children and Social Phobia

In order for someone younger than eighteen to be diagnosed with social phobia, the symptoms must last at least six months. The youth must be capable of having age-appropriate social relationships. The anxiety-provoking situations must be experienced in settings with peers and not only with adults.

Unlike adults, children do not have to have insight that their fear is unreasonable for the situation. When they do realize that their fear is not normal, they may try to conceal the problem. Children may also express their anxiety differently from the way adults express it. Children may express their anxiety through crying or temper tantrums. They may avoid social situations in which they will be with unfamiliar people.

GENERALIZED ANXIETY DISORDER

Generalized anxiety disorder (GAD) is characterized by excessive worry about everyday life. The types of worry differ from person to person and may focus on things from the past, present, or future. As with other disorders discussed here, the worry causes significant interference with daily functioning. Generalized anxiety disorder is often accompanied by somatic problems such as rapid heart rate, shortness of breath, chronic physical health problems, and gastric problems including nausea or diarrhea. People with GAD may also experience trembling, being easily startled, and substance abuse.

Diagnosing Generalized Anxiety Disorder

The criteria for GAD in the *DSM* include excessive anxiety and worry almost every day for at least six months that affects multiple different events or activities, as well as difficulty controlling the worry. Adults must meet both criteria, whereas children are required to meet only one. Three of the following symptoms (one for children) must also be present:

- Restlessness or feeling on edge
- Being easily fatigued
- Difficulty concentrating/mind going blank
- Irritability

- Muscle tension
- Sleep disturbance

Children and Generalized Anxiety Disorder

As stated above, children do not need to have as many of the symptoms of GAD as do adults in order to meet criteria for the diagnosis. Common worries experienced by children often focus on the health of their family or themselves, their level of competence in school or athletics, their past actions, and future events. The fears experienced are not realistic and are excessive for the child's developmental level. It is important for the mental health professional to evaluate whether the fears are based in reality. For example, a child about to have surgery may experience fear of dying. Once the surgery has passed, the fear will dissipate. In meeting the criteria for GAD, the child must have difficulty controlling worry, and daily functioning must be significantly impaired.

OBSESSIVE-COMPULSIVE DISORDER

Obsessive-compulsive disorder (OCD) is a very disruptive disorder prevalent in approximately 1 to 2 percent of the population, with 25 percent of those experiencing onset by age fourteen. Obsessive-compulsive disorder causes significant distress and frustration. It can be triggered by environmental or stressful factors, including normal developmental transitions such as starting school. When we think of OCD, we tend to think of people who have to wash their hands repeatedly before they can leave the bathroom, or those who turn the light switch on and off over and over. Youth with OCD experience excessive worry about bad things happening to themselves or someone they care about or become excessively preoccupied with something. The level of worry is far beyond a normal child's level of worry and is not usually related to anything realistic. These excessive intrusive thoughts or worries are called *obsessions*. Although obsessions can present around many different issues, some of the more common obsessions experienced by children and adolescents include the following:

- Constant worry that something is going to harm family or self
- Fear of germs or contamination
- Intrusive sounds or words

- Religious preoccupation
- Preoccupation with body wastes
- Intrusive thoughts related to sex or aggression

Trying to ignore or suppress an obsession only increases its intensity and the associated discomfort, which often leads to the development of compulsions. *Compulsions* are repetitive behaviors or mental acts that are performed to reduce the stress or prevent something bad from happening. They are excessive and usually not related to the situation to be avoided. They interfere with a person's functioning. The following compulsions are the most common among children and teens:

- Repeated hand washing, showering, or teeth brushing;
- Repeated rituals such as turning a light on and off a certain number of times before leaving a room;
- Repeatedly rechecking something, such as seeing if a door is locked;
- Having to touch an object over and over;
- Rituals to prevent harming self or others;
- Rituals of ordering or arranging things, such as ensuring that all the books on a bookshelf are perfectly aligned;
- Counting rituals such as counting to 100 before starting some task;
- Hoarding and collecting things;
- Cleaning rituals related to the house or other items.

The conduct of these rituals can take lots of patience on the part of families, caregivers, teachers, and others spending time with a youth. Trying to stop the youth from completing the ritual can result in serious behavior problems such as severe tantrums. A caregiver's failure to recognize the child's need to conduct rituals can also result in serious problems.

There are common signs that youth may be experiencing an obsession or compulsion. A youth's hands may be raw from constant washing or he or she may use a large amount of paper towels or soap. A caregiver may notice that a child's homework has holes in the paper due to excessive erasing or that a child is spending hours on homework but not completing it. Normal daily activities may take an exceptionally long time to complete, such as showers that take two hours each morning. Youth may voice fear of being contaminated and respond by refusing to eat a meal if someone touches their plate or food, for example. Children may refuse to leave the house for fear that something really bad will happen to their parent.

Obsessions and/or compulsions in a child or adolescent often result in isolation from others. They can become so intrusive that he or she does not have time to participate in life. Further, he or she will become isolated from friends and family due to the actual obsession or compulsion or the need to hide these symptoms from others and avoid the associated stigma.

Diagnosing Obsessive-Compulsive Disorder

To be diagnosed with OCD, a person must experience obsessions and/or compulsions that are time consuming and cause marked distress. These thoughts or rituals often interfere with daily functioning, resulting in a person missing work or being late to work, school, or appointments. In order to be diagnosed with OCD, adults must recognize that their obsessions or compulsions are excessive and not normal. The need to recognize the irrationality of thoughts and/or behaviors does not apply to children. Children do not have to recognize that their obsessions or compulsions are not normal; however, those who do recognize the irrationality may try to hide it from others.

POSTTRAUMATIC STRESS DISORDER

Posttraumatic stress disorder (PTSD) is a mental health disorder resulting from a traumatic event in the environment that changes a person's brain chemistry. It is often associated with veterans returning from war, and it is one of the most common mental health problems experienced by maltreated children. Children who have experienced severe physical abuse or domestic violence are at a high risk for developing PTSD. Because of the prevalence of PTSD in maltreated children, more attention will be focused on this disorder.

Posttraumatic stress disorder is a form of hyperarousal response, meaning that it is a state of increased mental and physiological tension. The response is the result of the brain's inability to process and store the memories of a traumatic event. Persons who develop PTSD have either experienced or witnessed some tragic event involving actual or threatened death or serious injury to themselves or someone else. They respond to the event with feelings of complete helplessness or intense fear and reexperience it in one of several ways. Reliving of the experience often occurs in flashbacks of the event. People may experience recurrent nightmares of the event or intrusive images or thoughts of the event. They may experience a sound, smell, sight, or feeling that reminds them of the event and causes a physiological response or intense distress psychologically.

Along with flashbacks or dreams of the event, other symptoms may include diminished interest or participation in significant activities, feelings of detachment or estrangement from others, restricted range of affect, difficulty falling or staying asleep, irritability or outbursts of anger, difficulty concentrating, hypervigilance, and exaggerated startle response (American Psychiatric Association, 2013).

Posttraumatic Stress Disorder and the Brain

Research studies on PTSD have found that persons with PTSD experience changes in their brain chemistry and functioning (Kandel, Schwartz, & Jessell, 2000; Perry, 2006; Solomon & Heide, 2005; Teicher et al., 2003; Van der Kolk, 1987). It has been found that adults with PTSD have increased heart rates and higher blood pressure than adults without PTSD. They also experience conditioned anxiety, agitation, and panic states. The majority of studies in the literature have been conducted with adults rather than with children. Psychophysiological studies on adults with PTSD have reported baseline autonomic activation as evidenced by increased heart rate, systolic blood pressure, and forehead electromyography. Other psychophysiological studies have found that adult PTSD patients have a more marked conditioned autonomic hyperactivity as well as conditioned anxiety, agitation, and panic states. High levels of catecholamines and their metabolites in plasma and urine suggest evidence of central and/or peripheral noradrenergic system dysfunction. Researchers have found altered receptor functioning of peripheral adrenergic receptors on platelets and lymphocytes and a significant decrease in number of platelet alpha-2 adrenergic receptors. Intact platelets are down regulated four times faster in PTSD patients than in other persons.

Posttraumatic stress disorder is considered a developmental disorder for children in that, as neurons are being developed and differentiated, damaging changes are occurring in the child's brain due to the changes and quantity of neurotransmitters resulting from trauma. These altered neurotransmitters thus alter the development of catecholamine receptor/effector systems and the functions mediated by them. Children who develop PTSD have alterations in the central and autonomic nervous systems, higher than normal levels of opiates in the brain, and an elevation of thyroid functioning. They have been found to excrete high levels of norepinephrine in urine, thus signifying a high level of circulating catecholamine. Evidence suggests that childhood trauma interferes with central nervous system maturation and causes lasting neurological changes. It is believed that some biochemical, functional, and structural changes in the brain are related to early and more chronic abuse and neglect that affect the process of brain development. Researchers have found that higher levels of exposure to violence result in more serious changes in the brains of children.

Two studies of childhood PTSD both found abnormal regulation of the simple autonomic nervous system mediated by catecholamine (Perry, 1994). The first study attempted to examine potential dysregulation of brainstem catecholamine by studying the platelet alpha-2 adrenergic receptors. A high correlation was found between resting heart rate and the density of platelet alpha-2 adrenergic receptors. Norepinephrine and epinephrine signal through alpha-2 adrenergic receptors in the central and peripheral nervous systems.

The second study compared heart rate changes for children with PTSD. A baseline heart rate was established for each child by measuring the heart rate while the child was sitting, followed by measuring the heart rate while the child was standing. The youth with PTSD were found to have a higher basal rate, meaning that they expended more energy in the body while standing than children without PTSD. Children with PTSD experienced either an overshoot of heart rate with a slow return to baseline or a normal increase in heart rate with a slow return to baseline. The combination of these two studies suggests poorly integrated brainstem function, increased sympathetic tone, and overreactive and poorly regulated brainstem catecholamine systems, meaning that brain development is significantly affected in children with PTSD.

Diagnosing Posttraumatic Stress Disorder

There are significant changes from the *DSM-IV* to the *DSM-5* for PTSD. In this book, following *DSM-IV* (American Psychiatric Association, 1994), we are including it with other anxious disorders. In the *DSM-5* (American Psychiatric

Association, 2013), PTSD is in a new chapter on trauma- and stressor-related disorders along with reactive attachment disorder, disinhibited social engagement disorder, acute stress disorder, and adjustment disorders. The disorders in this group are all characterized by exposure of a person to a catastrophic or aversive event followed by an expression of a clinical level of distress that may present itself in an internalized manner (anxiety or fear) or an externalized manner (anger or aggression).

The criteria for PTSD in the *DSM-5* remain very similar to those in the *DSM-IV*; however, the *DSM-5* changes the three diagnostic clusters to four clusters and changes some wording to be more sensitive to children and adolescents.

To be diagnosed with PTSD, a child must experience symptoms associated with PTSD for a month or longer, and these symptoms must cause significant problems in ability to function in normal activities and relationships. Following the traumatic event, the child must experience at least three symptoms related to persistently avoiding anything that may be associated with the trauma and have a general lack of responsiveness. In other words, as specified in the *DSM*, the child must present with at least three of the following symptoms:

- Avoidance of thoughts, feelings, or conversations associated with the trauma;
- Avoidance of activities, places, or people that arouse recollections of the trauma;
- Inability to recall an important aspect of the trauma;
- Markedly diminished interest or participation in significant activities;
- Feeling of detachment or estrangement from others;
- Restricted range of affect (e.g., does not expect to have a career, marriage, children, or a normal lifespan).

He or she must also experience persistent symptoms of increased arousal (not present before the trauma) as indicated by two (or more) of the following:

- Difficulty falling or staying asleep
- Irritability or outbursts of anger
- Difficulty concentrating
- Hypervigilance
- Exaggerated startle response

Children and Posttraumatic Stress Disorder

It can be difficult to diagnose PTSD in children due to the presentation of the symptoms. A child's symptoms may present similarly to those of another mental illness such as attention deficit hyperactivity disorder, conduct disorder, or bipolar disorder. The presentation of symptoms can also be different for children than for adults. For example, rather than having nightmares of the event, children commonly experience nightmares that are unrecognizable. Younger children may repetitively act out themes of the trauma in their play.

Assessment of PTSD in children necessitates a full psycho-social-emotional-biological evaluation across all areas of a child's life. The evaluation must include information from multiple persons involved in the child's life such as teachers, family members, coaches, or any others intimately involved with the child. Structured assessment instruments specific to the symptoms of PTSD in youth are also important to include in making the diagnosis.

The specific symptoms or disorders a child develops from maltreatment are based on the age of the child; the duration, extent, and level of abuse; the child's adaptive style; and other factors in the child's life such as emotional support received. Research on child maltreatment in PTSD has found that family history can affect the presentation of symptoms in childhood PTSD (Terr, 1991). For example, a child with a family history of schizophrenia has a higher likelihood of developing psychotic symptoms whereby the child loses touch with reality in response to maltreatment. The child may experience an inability to think clearly or understand reality, difficulty communicating effectively, or inability to behave appropriately, or he or she may respond to situations with exaggerated behaviors or with complete numbness.

A child whose family history includes anxiety disorders is more likely to develop symptoms of anxiety or an anxiety disorder, and a child with a family history of sociopathy and substance abuse is more likely to develop symptoms similar to conduct disorder. High rates of mental health problems and histories of trauma exposure and abuse have been found in adjudicated female youth. The variance in the presentation of symptoms makes identifying and treating PTSD in children very challenging. It is even more challenging in infants and children under the age of four because *DSM-IV* criteria are not sensitive enough to pick up PTSD in these younger children and infants. These young children often do not experience the hallmark features of adult PTSD, such as flashbacks and avoidance behaviors. Instead, symptoms of PTSD can be observed in a child's repetitive play in which he or she reenacts a traumatic theme. When reminders of the trauma occur, children often experience intense distress that can manifest itself as difficulty concentrating, disturbed sleep, irritability, or anger outbursts. Although less is known about children responding to maltreatment with dissociation, some children with PTSD will develop symptoms such as diminished interest in regular activities, blunted affect, listlessness, and/or detachment. Lack of understanding or recall of the trauma by the child adds to the difficulty.

SCREENING TOOLS FOR ANXIETY

There are many tools for screening or assessing for symptoms of anxiety. The instruments discussed below are just examples of existing tools. Although there are many others, these three have been tested and found to be valid and reliable for assessing anxiety in children. Some of these tools are completed by a clinician. Others are self-reports completed by the youth or caregiver reports completed by the caregiver about the child. None of these tools should be used as the sole criterion for diagnosing an anxiety disorder; however, they can be useful in screening for anxiety or for monitoring treatment effectiveness.

The Spence Children's Anxiety Scale

The Spence Children's Anxiety Scale (SCAS; Spence, Barrett, & Turner, 2003) is a tool used to assess the severity of anxiety symptoms across six anxiety domains (generalized anxiety, panic/agoraphobia, social phobia, separation anxiety, obsessive-compulsive disorder, and physical injury fears). The SCAS is available in three forms: youth self-report, caregiver report, and a caregiver preschool report. Each version of the scale takes about five to ten minutes to complete. Youth or the caregivers rate the frequency with which the youth experiences symptoms (*never*, *sometimes*, *often*, and *always*). The SCAS is sensitive to changes in symptoms; therefore, it is useful for monitoring the effectiveness of treatment. It has been translated into multiple languages. All versions of the scale are available free at http://www.scaswebsite.com.

Beck Anxiety Inventory for Youth

The Beck Anxiety Inventory for Youth (BYI) is a twenty-item self-report inventory for use with children and adolescents from seven to eighteen years old.

For each item, youth rate the frequency at which they experience a thought, feeling, or behavior related to anxiety from *never* to *always*. The BYI is used for screening, assessment, treatment planning, and measuring response to treatment. It takes approximately five to ten minutes for a youth to complete. It can be purchased online at http://www.pearsonclinical.com/psychology/products/1000 00153/beck-youth-inventories-second-edition-byiii.html?Pid = 015-8014-197 #tab-pricing.

Screen for Childhood Anxiety Related Disorders

Screen for Childhood Anxiety Related Disorders (SCARED) was developed to screen children and adolescents of ages eight and older for anxiety disorders (Birmaher et al., 1999). It consists of forty-one items that measure different types of anxiety based on the *DSM-IV* to include general anxiety, separation anxiety, social phobia, school phobia, and physical symptoms of anxiety. The youth is asked to rate each item as 0 = *not true*, 1 = *somewhat or sometimes true*, or 2 = *very true or often true*. A caregiver report form is also available. The form takes approximately five minutes to complete. It can be downloaded free from http://www.wpic.pitt.edu/research under tools and assessments.

CASE STUDIES

Here are some case studies of youth who experience some form of anxiety (names have been changed). In the next chapter, we will discuss evidence-based treatments and practices used to treat anxiety in children and adolescents. We will return to each of these youths to discuss the diagnoses, the different interventions they received, and the outcomes.

Andrea

Andrea was seven when she was placed in foster care. She was removed from her mother because the mother's boyfriend was physically and sexually abusing her and her mother was unable to protect her. Prior to the boyfriend moving into the home, Andrea was an average student. She was pleasant and got along well with her peers. One of her teachers made a report to Child Welfare Services because she noticed that Andrea had started coming to school with bruises on her body and had a significant change in her schoolwork and behaviors. Andrea became irritable and angry with her peers, often without provocation. She stopped doing her homework and in class she seemed to daydream rather than pay attention.

Andrea was placed in a home with three other foster children. She shared a room with another little girl. In the foster home, she continued to be irritable. She hardly interacted with the other children or her foster parents. She did not seem to have any interest in normal childhood activities. If someone walked up behind Andrea, she jumped. At night, she would wake up screaming as a result of having nightmares about her mother's boyfriend trying to find her and kill her.

Consider the following questions:

1. What symptoms was Andrea experiencing?

2. Based on the information provided, does she meet the criteria for an anxiety disorder? Explain. If she does which one?

3. Based on your current knowledge, what interventions would you suggest? Do you believe that she received the appropriate intervention or treatment?

4. Who should be included in Andrea's treatment planning and interventions?

5. What barriers might get in the way of effectively intervening with Andrea?

6. What suggestions/thoughts/ideas do you have for the other members of Andrea's family?

Juan

Juan is a fourteen-year-old who was really late getting to school nearly every day of the week. Each morning before Juan left his house, he was compelled to count to 100 over and over for fear that something bad would happen to him if he did not. When Juan tried to ignore his thoughts and not count, he became more anxious and ended up having to count to 100 more times than usual. The same thing would happen if his mother tried to get him to leave the house on time to get to school. His mother did not know about his counting ritual. To her, it seemed that Juan was being resistant to going to school and not following her directions. She took Juan to the community mental health clinic for evaluation.

Try to answer the following questions:

1. What symptoms was Juan experiencing?

2. Based on the information provided, does he meet the criteria for an anxious disorder? Explain. If he does, which one?

3. Based on your current knowledge, what interventions would you suggest?

4. Who should be included in Juan's treatment planning and interventions?

5. What barriers might get in the way of effectively intervening with Juan?

6. What suggestions/thoughts/ideas do you have for the other members of Juan's family?

Andy

Andy is a six-year-old. He is a very bright child. However, whenever he walked into a building, any building, he felt compelled to go into each restroom and touch the pipes under the sink. As can be imagined, this could take a considerable amount of time and was very embarrassing to his parents. It got to the point where they would not take him anywhere. He was either at school or at home. A doctor recommended putting Andy on medication to control his compulsions. Neither of his parents was comfortable with their son taking meds. They felt that it would be better to let him grow out of it.

When Andy went to school each day, he had to touch all the sink pipes before he went to his classroom. He was consistently late to class. His mother started driving him to school an hour early every day so he could complete his ritual before class started. It became a huge issue that Andy had to check the pipes in the girls' restroom and the teacher and staff restrooms, as well as the boys' restroom. At first, the school was very tolerant about Andy's need, but as he got older, the school did not feel that it was appropriate for him to go into the girls' and teachers' restrooms. They tried to stop Andy, which resulted in a huge anger outburst. His parents ended up removing him from school and home schooling him. Andy became very isolated in his home.

Can you answer the following questions?

1. What symptoms was Andy experiencing?
2. Based on the information provided, does he meet the criteria for an anxious disorder? Explain. If he does, which one?
3. Based on your current knowledge, what interventions would you suggest?
4. Who should be included in Andy's treatment planning and interventions?
5. What barriers might get in the way of effectively intervening with Andy?
6. What suggestions/thoughts/ideas do you have for the other members of Andy's family?

Reggie

Reggie is a fifteen-year-old high school student. Reggie refused to attend any events such as dances or parties because he was afraid that he would do or say something embarrassing. When teachers asked him questions in front of the class, his face turned red. He would not answer the teacher's question for fear of not giving the correct answer or saying something stupid. Reggie even missed school on days when he was supposed to do a presentation in front of the class and instead accepted an F for the assignment. He felt that he was not as smart as the other students.

Consider the following questions.

1. What symptoms was Reggie experiencing?
2. Based on the information provided, does he meet the criteria for an anxious disorder? Explain. If he does, which one?
3. Based on your current knowledge, what interventions would you suggest?
4. Who should be included in Reggie's treatment planning and interventions?

5. What barriers might get in the way of effectively intervening with Reggie?

6. What suggestions/thoughts/ideas do you have for the other members of Reggie's family?

REFERENCES

American Psychiatric Association. (1994). *Diagnostic and statistical manual of mental disorders* (4th ed.). Washington, DC: Author.

American Psychiatric Association. (2013). *Diagnostic and statistical manual of mental disorders* (5th ed.). Washington, DC: Author.

Birmaher, B., Brent, D. A., Chiappetta, L., Bridge, J., Monga, S., & Baugher, M. (1999). Psychometric properties of the Screen for Child Anxiety Related Emotional Disorders (SCARED): A replication study. *Journal of the American Academy of Child and Adolescent Psychiatry, 38*, 1230–1236.

Kandel, E. R., Schwartz, J. H., & Jessell, T. M. (2000). *Principles of neural science* (4th ed.). New York: McGraw-Hill.

Perry, B. D. (1994). Neurobiological sequelae of childhood trauma: Post-traumatic stress disorders in children. In M. Murburg (Ed.), *Catecholamine function in posttraumatic stress disorder: Emerging concepts*. Washington, DC: American Psychiatric Press.

Perry, B. D. (2006). Applying principles of neurodevelopment of clinical work with maltreated and traumatized children: The neurosequential model of therapeutics. In N. B. Webb (Ed.), *Working with traumatized youth in child welfare* (pp. 27–52). New York: Guilford Press.

Solomon, E. P., & Heide, K. M. (2005). The biology of trauma: Implications for treatment. *Journal of Interpersonal Violence, 20*, 51–60.

Spence, S. H., Barrett, P. M., & Turner, C. M. (2003). Psychometric properties of the Spence Children's Anxiety Scale with young adolescents. *Journal of Anxiety Disorders, 17*, 605–625.

Teicher, M. H., Anderson, S. L., Polcari, A., Anderson, C. M., Navalta, C. P., & Kim, D. M. (2003). The neurobiological consequences of early stress and childhood maltreatment. *Neuroscience and Biobehavioral Reviews, 27*, 33–44.

Terr, L. C. (1991). Childhood traumas: An outline and overview. *American Journal of Psychiatry, 148*, 10–20.

Van der Kolk, B. A. (1987). The separation cry and the trauma response: Developmental issues in the psychobiology of attachment and separation. In B. A. Van der Kolk (Ed.), *Psychological trauma*. Washington, DC: American Psychiatric Press.

CHAPTER 7

Treatment of Anxiety Disorders

THE TREATMENT of anxiety disorders is very similar to the treatment of depression. As with depression, anxiety is treated with psychotropic medications, various psychotherapies, or a combination of both. Evidence-based interventions and practices for treating the different types of anxiety utilize cognitive-behavioral therapy (CBT) techniques such as teaching youth how negative thinking affects levels of anxiety, how to identify the physical aspects of anxiety, and how to change thoughts or use relaxation techniques to reduce anxiety. Unless children or adolescents are a danger to themselves or others or significantly unable to function, psychotherapy is often the preferred first line of treatment. If after a few weeks psychotherapy is ineffective, medication is added to the treatment regimen.

MEDICATION TREATMENT

Medications used to treat anxiety disorder include

antianxiety medications and antidepressants. The most frequently prescribed antidepressants used in the treatment of anxiety are in the selective serotonin reuptake inhibitor (SSRI) class. These include Prozac, Zoloft, Lexapro, Paxil, and Celexa (see chapter 5 for a full discussion of antidepressants). Both Zoloft and Paxil are approved by the U.S. Food and Drug Administration (FDA) for treating generalized anxiety disorder (GAD). Effexor, a serotonin norepinephrine reuptake inhibitor (SNRI), has been found effective in treating obsessive-compulsive disorder. Antidepressants used to treat anxiety in youth come with the same black box warnings (the most serious medication warnings given by the FDA) as they do for treating depression due to the possibility that they may cause suicidal thoughts. Therefore, it is important to closely monitor any young person taking an antidepressant. Four to six weeks should be allowed to experience the full effect of the medications.

Another class of medications used to treat anxiety is the benzodiazepines (see Table 7.1). This class of drugs affects the central nervous system by enhancing the response of receptors in the brain to a neurotransmitter called gamma-aminobutyric acid (GABA), thereby negatively charging the neuron and making it resistant to excitation. Benzodiazepines are rarely used in treating anxiety disorders in youth because they have the potential for dependence. However, they are occasionally used to treat extreme levels of anxiety on a very short-term basis.

Some of the most commonly prescribed benzodiazepines are Klonopin, used mostly for treating social phobia and GAD; Ativan, used mostly for panic disorder; and Xanax, which is used for both panic disorder and GAD. A benefit of

Table 7.1. Benzodiazepines for treating anxiety

Brand name	Generic name
Ativan	Lorazepam
Dalmane	Flurazepam
Klonopin	Clonazepam
Halcion	Triazolam
Librium	Chlordiazepoxide
Restoril	Temazepam
Serax	Oxazepam
Tranxene	Clorazepate
Valium	Diazepam
Xanax	Alprazolam

using benzodiazepines on a short-term basis is their relatively few side effects. The main side effects experienced by children and adolescents are drowsiness, sedation, and decreased mental acuity.

PSYCHOTHERAPIES AND ANXIETY

There are several manualized and non-manualized evidence-based practices and treatments for anxiety. Most of the evidence-based interventions are based on a combination of cognitive-behavioral, trauma, and social learning theories. Many of the interventions focus treatment on both the youth and the caregiver(s). Empirically supported practices focus on helping the youth identify negative thinking that leads to anxiety and learning new skills to manage it. For caregivers, many of the interventions focus on education about anxiety and the role problematic parenting styles can play in the youth's anxiety level. Caregivers are taught more effective ways of parenting. Some examples of existing evidence-based treatments are discussed in the following subsections.

Coping Cat

There are several manualized interventions based on cognitive-behavioral theory. Coping Cat is one example of a manualized cognitive-behavioral intervention for children from ages eight to seventeen (Kendall, Choudhury, Hudson, & Webb, 2002; Kendall & Hedtke, 2006a, 2006b). The intervention consists of sixteen sessions. These sessions focus on teaching youth about anxiety, helping them identify stress-inducing situations, and helping them develop coping skills. Coping Cat uses techniques common to CBT such as role playing, relaxation training, self-reinforcement techniques, and practicing skills in real life situations to help the youth develop the skills necessary for managing anxiety.

Once youth are able to identify the physical reactions related to the onset of anxiety, they can learn ways to manage the anxiety before it reaches a serious point. Youth are also taught to identify thinking errors (faulty beliefs) that lead to anxious feelings in order to change negative cognitions to more positive ones. The last eight sessions focus on practicing the new skills, first in imaginary stress-inducing situations, and then working up to practicing the skills in real life stress-inducing situations as appropriate. This method is a form of an effective stress management technique called systematic desensitization.

Trauma-Focused Cognitive-Behavioral Therapy

Trauma-focused cognitive-behavioral therapy (TF-CBT) is an evidence-based intervention appropriate for treating children and adolescents who have experienced abuse, neglect, or other traumatic experience or witnessed a traumatic event. Many adults believe that children are resilient and able to forget traumatic events. Rather than understanding the negative consequences of trauma, they have expectations of the child and how the child should behave. Research has found that young children are negatively affected by traumatic events and need a way to derive meaning from them. Trauma-focused CBT has been found effective in treating posttraumatic stress disorder. It is based on learning, behavioral, and cognitive theories. Using techniques of CBT and family therapies, treatment focuses on both the youth and a non-offending caregiver with emphasis on improving attachment and communication between them. Like CBT, TF-CBT is time limited, lasting twelve to eighteen sessions.

The key components of TF-CBT have been summarized by the mnemonic PRACTICE (Substance Abuse and Mental Health Services Administration, 2014):

- The *P* stands for psychoeducation and parenting skills. This component of treatment focuses on educating caregivers about the effects of abuse and trauma on children because caregivers who do not have this understanding often set unrealistic expectations of how their child should feel and behave. Research has found that problematic parenting styles contribute to a youth's anxiety. Caregivers who are overly protective often set limits on their children that are excessively restrictive and do not allow the children to experience developmentally appropriate situations in which to experience new situations and develop coping skills. Caregivers who have difficulty coping with their own anxiety model ineffective ways of coping for their children. Caregivers are taught more effective parenting skills, effective communication skills, and how to respond empathetically to their child's feelings.
- *R* stands for relaxation techniques. Relaxation techniques are one of the most effective ways to manage stress and anxiety. Young people, especially younger children, feel a sense of accomplishment and empowerment through learning and using these techniques. Using a

relaxation technique called progressive muscle relaxation, youth learn to isolate their focus onto different parts of the body, to tense the muscles in that area, and to then release all the tension. This continues until the entire body feels relaxed. Focused breathing is a relaxation technique that helps a youth take long, deep breaths and relax the body more and more with each exhale. Visual imagery is another effective relaxation technique in which youth close their eyes and focus on being in a safe, comfortable environment such as lying in a meadow with the sun beaming down or floating on a magic carpet.

- *A* is for affective expression and regulation. The therapist works with both the child and caregiver to manage emotional reactions to places or situations that are reminders of the abuse. Rather than reacting in a destructive manner, they learn to identify and express their emotions verbally and to self-soothe.

- Cognitive coping and processing (*C*) are taught to the youth and caregiver so that they connect their thoughts with their feelings and behaviors. The therapist helps them identify faulty beliefs (thinking errors) that result in unconstructive behaviors and methods of coping. They learn to reframe thinking errors with positive thoughts that will then lead to more positive behaving and coping.

- *T* stands for trauma narrative and processing. Developing a trauma narrative is a key component in helping youth cope with their trauma. The therapeutic environment provides a safe place for children to process their experiences and make sense of the traumatic event(s). They can confront upsetting thoughts and feelings resulting from the event. When developing a trauma narrative, a therapist guides the caregiver and child through a series of questions to help them recreate the traumatic event(s) in some way. Young children often recreate the traumatic event through play or artwork.

- In vivo exposure (*I*), also known as systematic desensitization (as discussed previously), is another key component of TF-CBT. After the youth learns coping and relaxation techniques, the therapist begins exposing him or her to places or situations that are reminders of the trauma, such as the room where the trauma took place. The therapist may first help the youth visualize the stress-inducing place or situation while helping him or her to practice the new coping and relaxation techniques. Once the youth is able to manage emotional reactions while visualizing the place or situation, the therapist will gradually bring him or her closer and closer until he or she is able to manage emotional reactions when fully exposed to the stress-inducing place or situation.

- The final two letters, *C* and *E*, stand for conjoint parent/child sessions and enhancing personal safety and future growth. During conjoint sessions, youths are able to share their trauma narrative with the caregiver. These joint sessions provide opportunities to normalize the anxiety experienced by the child. The caregiver learns the skills needed to provide positive affect and to encourage the child. The family learns skills to improve communication with each other. The final key component of TF-CBT is education and training to maintain the safety of the youth. Non-offending caregivers are taught the skills needed to help their children develop the sense of safety that is important for overcoming anxiety. They learn to identify and avoid situations that could put their children in danger of abuse. Youth are taught skills that empower them to look after their personal safety as well.

Child-Parent Psychotherapy

Child-parent psychotherapy (CPP) is an empirically supported intervention aimed at treating very young children, from birth through age six, who have experienced at least one traumatic event resulting in emotional, behavioral, and/or attachment problems (National Child Traumatic Stress Network, 2007). The overarching goal of CPP is to strengthen the attachment between child and caregiver(s) and return the child to a normal developmental path. This intervention has been evaluated and found effective across racially and ethnically diverse populations.

Child-parent psychotherapy is not a manualized intervention. Therefore, it can be more difficult to learn than some of the other empirically supported interventions. Clinicians providing CPP are usually master's level social workers or psychologists with specialized training in mental health issues. In order to provide CPP, a clinician must receive face-to-face training and become certified as a CPP provider. For the certified CPP clinician, ongoing phone consultation and occasional booster sessions help increase fidelity to the model and provide support and guidance for dealing with difficult situations.

Child-parent psychotherapy is a didactic intervention based on attachment theory, and drawing also from psychodynamic, trauma, social learning, and cognitive-behavioral theories. Treatment includes key components of TF-CBT. During sessions, caregivers learn about the effects of trauma on behavior and functioning and how to respond empathetically and give their child positive affect. For example, a session might consist of a child playing while the therapist/counselor teaches the caregiver to pay attention to the child's play and respond in empathetic, supportive ways. When the child is very young, such as an infant, treatment focuses on providing the caregiver with the skills needed to provide a safe and loving environment. If caregivers have their own unresolved trauma issues, they are addressed in separate sessions with the caregiver.

CASE STUDIES

Andrea

Andrea is the seven-year-old who was placed in foster care because she had been physically and sexually abused by her mother's boyfriend and her mother had been unable to protect her. Andrea was placed in a foster home where three other foster children lived. She isolated herself from the other children. She continued to isolate herself and did not participate in activities or develop any friendships in her new school. She continued to have nightmares and started wetting the bed. The foster family was at a loss as to how to manage Andrea. They requested that she be removed from their home. Andrea was put into another foster home with foster parents who had been trained to manage children with emotional or behavioral problems. Child Protective Services paid for her to attend counseling with a therapist trained in TF-CBT. She was diagnosed with posttraumatic stress disorder.

The therapist asked to have Andrea's mother participate in the therapy sessions. Child Protective Services allowed the mother to participate and the mother agreed. She wanted to have Andrea return home and broke up with her boyfriend. Near the end of treatment, both the mother and Andrea had made great progress. The therapist advocated for Andrea to spend increasing increments of time at home to test how the two would do together. The therapist, case worker, mother, and Andrea met to develop a treatment plan that led to Andrea returning home to live. After Andrea spent six months at home, the Child Protective Services case was closed.

Juan

Juan is the fourteen-year-old who was really late getting to school nearly every day of the week. He could not leave his house until he had counted to 100 over and over for fear that something bad would happen to him if he did not. When Juan tried to ignore his thoughts and not count, he became more anxious and ended up having to count to 100 more times than usual. Juan's mother became frustrated with him and took him to the community mental health clinic for evaluation. Juan was evaluated by a psychiatrist, who diagnosed him with obsessive-compulsive disorder and started him on a low dose of the medication Effexor. Within two weeks, Juan's counting ritual had subsided considerably. Within four weeks, the ritual had ceased and Juan began to function better in school.

Andy

Andy is the six-year-old who felt compelled to go into each restroom in any building he entered and touch the pipes under the sink. His parents took him to a doctor who recommended medication. They refused to put him on medication. His compulsion resulted in problems in school that eventually led to his parent's homeschooling him and his becoming very isolated. Andy got to the point where he would not leave his house. If his parents tried to make him leave, he became very upset and screamed and yelled until his parents usually gave up and left him at home alone, even though he was so young. One evening when his parents were not home, Andy played with matches and set his bed on fire. The fire spread quickly. A neighbor saw smoke and called 911. When the firefighters arrived, they found Andy home alone and standing in the doorway crying. His room was completely burned, but he was not harmed. Child Protective Services was called.

Andy was allowed to stay with his parents as long as they agreed not to leave him alone and to participate in family therapy. His parents agreed. The therapist provided services in the family's home. They met with the therapist twice a week for an hour each time. The therapist diagnosed Andy with anxiety disorder not otherwise specified, meaning that he clearly had an anxiety disorder, but did not meet the criteria for obsessive-compulsive disorder. The therapist provided Andy with CBT. Andy got to the point where he could leave the house. He learned to cope with and control the need to touch all the bathroom pipes in a building and was able to start leaving the house and going places with his family. He was discharged from therapy and the Child Protective Services case was closed. It is not known if he ever returned to school or participated in age-appropriate activities with peers.

Reggie

Reggie is the fourteen-year-old who refused to attend any events such as dances or parties because he was afraid that he would do or say something embarrassing. He did not have any friends and began to exhibit symptoms of depression. He was diagnosed with social phobia and began CBT. He became less anxious, but still had difficulty interacting with others and seemed depressed. After five weeks in counseling, his counselor referred him to a psychiatrist. The psychiatrist put him on the antidepressant Paxil. After a month on Paxil, Reggie was significantly less anxious and less depressed. The therapist continued to work with him and encouraged Andy to join the youth group at his church, which Andy did. He began to participate in church activities and developed some friendships. He began to feel more confident in school and stopped avoiding situations where he would be the center of attention, such as answering questions in class.

Study Questions

1. What do these real life scenarios have in common?
2. What are the differences?
3. Now that you have learned what happened to each of the youths, do you have any different thoughts about how you would have handled the situation if you were the families' social worker?

REFERENCES

Kendall, P. C., Choudhury, M., Hudson, J., & Webb, A. (2002). *The CAT project manual for the cognitive-behavioral treatment of anxious adolescents.* Ardmore, PA: Workbook Publishing.
Kendall, P. C., & Hedtke, K. (2006a). *Cognitive-behavioral therapy for anxious children: Therapist manual* (3rd ed.). Ardmore, PA: Workbook Publishing.

Kendall, P. C., & Hedtke, K. (2006b). *The Coping CAT workbook* (2nd ed.). Ardmore, PA: Workbook Publishing.

National Child Traumatic Stress Network. (2007). *Child parent psychotherapy fact sheet.* Retrieved from http://www.nctsn.org/nctsn_assets/pdfs/promising_practices/Child _Parent_Psychotherapy_CPP_fact_sheet_3-20-07.pdf

Substance Abuse and Mental Health Services Administration. (2014). *National registry of evidence-based programs and practices: Trauma-focused cognitive-behavioral therapy (TF-CBT).* Retrieved from http://www.nrepp.samhsa.gov/viewinter vention.aspx?id = 135

CHAPTER 8

Attention Deficit Hyperactivity Disorder

Attention deficit hyperactivity disorder (ADHD) affects as many as 1 in 20 children (National Institute of Mental Health, 2012). It affects both boys and girls, but it is more predominant in boys, with a prevalence rate three to four times higher. Attention deficit hyperactivity disorder is characterized by inattention, hyperactivity, and impulsivity. The behaviors experienced are more severe and occur more frequently than would be expected for the developmental level of the child. The impulsive and hyperactive behaviors and inattentiveness impede a youth's success in school, relationships with peers, and family relationships.

Some children experience inattentiveness, some experience hyperactive or impulsive behaviors, and others experience a combination of both hyperactive/impulsive behavior and inattentiveness. Inattentiveness can interfere with a youth's ability to complete tasks such as homework or activities that require focus for some period of time. Children who experience problems with impulsiveness often get in trouble for doing things spontaneously. They may experience multiple trips to an emergency room for accidents related to inattentiveness or risky behavior associated with their impulsiveness. The effects of ADHD on the lives of those who experience it and those around them will be discussed further in this chapter.

CAUSES

The exact causes of ADHD are not yet known. Prior to technologies such as magnetic resonance imaging (MRI), ADHD was thought to be caused by environmental factors, with inconsistent parenting being commonly blamed. Current research is focused on possible linkages between ADHD and biological, genetic, environmental, and nutritional causes (National Institute of Mental Health, 2012). In the area of nutrition, the general public has commonly believed that giving children too much sugar makes them hyperactive and causes ADHD. Researchers have conducted extensive research on the correlation between sugar and ADHD. To date, there has been no evidence that links sugar to ADHD. Giving a child too much sugar does not cause ADHD (Millichap & Yee, 2012). Most recently research has emerged identifying food additives as a cause or contributor in the development of ADHD. As with sugar, there is no empirical evidence to support food additives as a cause or contributor to ADHD (Nigg, Lewis, Edinger, & Falk, 2012). Research on possible connections between nutrition and ADHD continues to be a focus.

Environmental factors being studied as possible causes or contributors to the development of ADHD include exposure to high levels of lead and in utero exposure to cigarette smoke and alcohol. There is some evidence suggesting that children exposed to high levels of lead, found in the paint of old buildings, experience higher risks of developing ADHD than other children (Millichap, 2008). There is also empirical evidence suggesting that children born to mothers who drank alcohol or smoked cigarettes while pregnant experience a higher prevalence of ADHD (Froehlich et al., 2009; Nomura, Marks, & Halperin, 2010).

Genetics research has found a familial link to ADHD (Faraone & Mick, 2010; Gizer, Ficks, & Waldman, 2009). Twin studies have found that ADHD tends to run in families. Children with a parent, uncle, or grandparent with ADHD are more likely to develop ADHD than a child with no familial history.

Researchers are currently studying several genes that have been identified as possible contributors to ADHD. Researchers hope that identifying genes that cause ADHD will allow treatments to be targeted specifically to those genes prior to the onset of ADHD, thus preventing its onset.

ATTENTION DEFICIT HYPERACTIVITY DISORDER AND THE BRAIN

Researchers are actively studying delays and abnormalities in brain development of youth with ADHD (see, for example, Gilliam et al., 2011, and Shaw et al., 2012). Research on the brain has found that children diagnosed with ADHD experience normal brain development, but the development in the frontal cortex is delayed on average by three years (Shaw, Eckstrand, et al., 2007). This area of the brain plays a part in cognitive functioning related to the ability to control impulsive behavior, focus attention, make sound judgments, solve problems, and exhibit socially appropriate behaviors.

Another part of the brain, the motor cortex, has been found to mature faster than normal in children with ADHD. The motor cortex is involved in the planning, control, and execution of actions and behavior. There is some belief that differences in the development of the frontal and motor cortexes play a role in the restlessness and fidgetiness that accompanies ADHD.

Other studies on the brain have found that children with ADHD who carry a particular version of a gene that is responsible for brain development have thinner brain tissue in areas of the brain responsible for controlling attention. As they move into puberty, the brain tissue becomes normal and the symptoms of ADHD improve (Shaw, Gornick, et al., 2007). Youth with this particular version of the gene have been found to have higher IQ and better clinical outcomes than youth with other versions of the same gene.

DIAGNOSING ATTENTION DEFICIT HYPERACTIVITY DISORDER

As with all other mental health disorders, ADHD is diagnosed following a thorough psychosocial evaluation and after ruling out other plausible causes for the symptoms. A thorough physical is important to rule out health problems such as seizures, problems with vision, inner ear infections, or other health problems that interfere with thought processes or behaviors and that could better account for the problems.

There are notable changes from the *DSM-IV* (American Psychiatric Association, 1994) to the *DSM-5* (American Psychiatric Association, 2013) for diagnosing ADHD. The *DSM-5* reports on presentation of symptoms rather than identifying a subtype of ADHD. During the development of the *DSM-5*, the workgroup concluded from the empirical literature that types of ADHD are not stable over time (Lahey, Pelham, Loney, Lee, & Willcutt, 2005); therefore, reporting on the presentation of the symptoms was more appropriate (Castellanos, 2011). The *DSM-IV* specified the criteria for each subtype. A person was required to exhibit at least six symptoms of inattention (see Table 8.1) to be diagnosed with predominantly inattentive type, or six symptoms of hyperactive/impulsive behavior (see Tables 8.2 and 8.3) for predominantly hyperactive-impulsive type, or to meet criteria for both inattentive and hyperactive-impulsive types for the combined type. According to *DSM-5* criteria, a person is diagnosed

Table 8.1. Symptoms of inattention

• Often does not give close attention to details or makes careless mistakes in schoolwork, work, or other activities;
• Often has trouble keeping attention on tasks or play activities;
• Often does not seem to listen when spoken to directly;
• Often does not follow instructions and fails to finish schoolwork, chores, or duties in the workplace (not due to oppositional behavior or failure to understand instructions);
• Often has trouble organizing activities;
• Often avoids, dislikes, or doesn't want to do things that take a lot of mental effort for a long period of time (such as schoolwork or homework);
• Often loses things needed for tasks and activities (e.g., toys, school assignments, pencils, books, or tools);
• Is often easily distracted;
• Is often forgetful in daily activities.

Table 8.2. Symptoms of hyperactivity-impulsivity

• Often fidgets with hands or feet or squirms in seat;
• Often gets up from seat when remaining in seat is expected;
• Often runs about or climbs when and where it is not appropriate (adolescents or adults may feel very restless);
• Often has trouble playing or enjoying leisure activities quietly;
• Often on the go or often acts as if driven by a motor;
• Often talks excessively.

Table 8.3. Symptoms of impulsivity

• Often blurts out answers before questions have been finished;
• Often has trouble waiting for a turn;
• Often interrupts or intrudes on others (e.g., butts into conversations or games).

with ADHD and then a specifier is added to define the symptoms: predominantly inattentive, hyperactive, impulsive, or a combination of all three.

The *DSM-IV* required symptoms to be evident by the age of seven. The age by which symptoms are required increased to twelve years old in the *DSM-5* (Kieling et al., 2010). The *DSM-IV* required symptoms to persist for at least six months across two or more settings (i.e., home, school, and work) and to cause significant functional impairment. The *DSM-5* workgroup recognized that parents are not good informants of their child's behavior while in school; therefore, the *DSM-5* suggests that clinicians obtain information from more than one adult source (Castellanos, 2011). The ADHD workgroup pulled back from requiring two informants because it would be costly and time consuming for clinicians. To determine if a person fully meets all the criteria, assessment includes investigation across life domains and seeks to determine if the home, school, work, or other environment is unusually stressful; how the person functions across settings; the duration, frequency, and context of symptoms; and the appropriateness of behaviors for the developmental age of the person.

The *DSM-5* no longer excludes a person with an intellectual or developmental disability from being diagnosed with ADHD. In reviewing the literature, the workgroup concluded that there is clear evidence that ADHD and autism spectrum disorders are commonly comorbid with one another (Castellanos, 2011).

CHILDREN, ADOLESCENTS, AND ATTENTION DEFICIT HYPERACTIVITY DISORDER

Symptoms of ADHD usually appear between the ages of three and six, but often go undiagnosed until children first begin school, which is the first time they are expected to remain in their seat, focus on tasks, and follow rules throughout the day. It is often teachers who first notice the symptoms because the child has trouble following rules, has difficulty with completing tasks, or seems to space out. Attention deficit hyperactivity disorder is the most common reason for children, particularly boys, to be referred to a mental health professional. Referral is due to the disruption that can go along with the impulsive behavior and the short attention span associated with the disorder.

Youth with inattentive symptoms are easily distracted. A noise in another room or in the school hall can easily distract their attention from tasks. Classrooms with lots of decorations can be very distracting. These youth have difficulty maintaining focus on people talking to them. They may appear to be daydreaming. Rapid processing of information and following directions are very challenging. Faced with a request involving compound instructions, a twelve-year-old child experiencing ADHD may have difficulty processing the information and following through with the task. For instance, twelve-year-old children without ADHD who were told to pick up their toys, take them to their room, and put them where they belong would be able to process the information and follow through with the request. A child with ADHD might not be able to process the information and therefore might not complete all of the tasks. Adults may incorrectly associate their behavior with oppositional defiant disorder.

Youth with ADHD who predominantly experience symptoms of inattention may go undiagnosed. They are not disruptive in class and can get along with other children. Teachers and parents may feel that they lack initiative to do well in school or that they are lazy. The ADHD is overlooked because we typically picture a hyperactive child when we think of ADHD. Inattention can fly under the radar.

Youth experiencing hyperactive symptoms have difficulty sitting still, appearing to be in constant motion. They tend to squirm in their seats or have to continually stand up. They talk nonstop and seem to get into everything around them. They have trouble waiting to take their turn in games, waiting in line for a drink at a water fountain, or waiting to get their lunch. They become bored easily and jump from one activity to another, not being able to focus for more than a few minutes on any task that is not enjoyable, making it very difficult for them to complete tasks. They have difficulty focusing on details and turn in sloppy or incomplete work. Without structure and help, they forget things, such as to complete their homework or to take it back to school. Children experiencing hyperactivity and impulsiveness can also be overlooked as they may be thought to have a behavioral problem and just lack discipline.

Dealing with a child who has ADHD can be very challenging and requires a significant amount of patience. It can be frustrating to have a child or student who exhibits challenging behaviors without considering consequences or shows emotions without restraint. It can be very difficult for the youth with ADHD as well. Because of their impulsive behaviors, other kids may not want to play with them, leaving them to become isolated and left out of pro-social activities. Getting in trouble constantly for not sitting still, blurting out answers, or exhibiting other problem behaviors during school can result in constant trips to the principal. The problem is not that they do not want to follow rules; following rules is often beyond their control.

Being unsuccessful in school and unable to make good grades can be another source of frustration for children with ADHD. Approximately 40 to 60 percent of youth with ADHD have co-occurring learning disabilities. Others have normal or above normal IQs, but still struggle in school due to their symptoms. Both have the potential of failing classes or entire grades. Self-esteem can be significantly damaged. Youth end up being disciplined for making bad grades and told that they are just not trying hard enough. All of these negatives in their lives can result in depression, drug or alcohol abuse, or developing relationships with oppositional-defiant or antisocial peer groups.

CASE STUDIES

Following are some case studies for youth experiencing disorders similar to those discussed in this chapter. Following each case study is a list of questions for review. In the next chapter, we will explore evidence-based treatments and practices for ADHD. We will return to the case studies presented in this chapter to learn of the actual types of interventions provided to these youths.

Eric

Eric is a ten-year-old boy living with his grandmother. Before he came to live with her at age seven, his grandmother reported that he was removed from his mother's care by Child Protective Services as a result of physical abuse. Eric had no contact with his father or his father's family. Child Protective Services allowed his mother to visit as long as his grandmother was present.

Eric had significant difficulty in school. He was antsy and could not remain seated. He refused to do his schoolwork, and he did not get along with the other children. He did not have any friends and did not participate in any activities with other kids. By the age of ten, he had been kicked out of two elementary schools, the last one for stabbing another student with a pencil.

Eric's grandmother took him to a community mental health center when he moved in with her. She reported that he had tried to hang himself twice, had killed a puppy, and was all over the place. Eric received medication for ADHD and depression and attended counseling once a week. His grandmother met with the therapist at the end of every appointment to give an update on his week. Each week for nearly three years, Eric's grandmother reported that he continued to be out of control and to experience episodes. When his counselor tried to talk with Eric about his mother and his suicide attempts, all he would say is that he did not remember. When asked about why he continued to have episodes at home, he would say something negative about himself.

Consider the following questions:

1. What symptoms was Eric experiencing?

2. Does he meet the criteria for a diagnosis of any of the types of ADHD? Explain. If he does, which type?

3. Based on your current knowledge, what interventions would you suggest? Do you believe that the appropriate intervention or treatment was provided?

4. Who should be included in the treatment planning and interventions?

5. What barriers might get in the way of effectively intervening?

6. What suggestions/thoughts/ideas do you have for the other members of his family?

Peter

When Peter was twelve years old and in the seventh grade, he had difficulty focusing in class. He was failing all of his classes and tested below his grade level on standardized tests. In class, Peter was the class clown. He constantly made jokes and did things to make classmates laugh. He would not remain seated. When teachers tried to redirect him, he became oppositional. He was sent to the office for his behaviors and for disturbing class on a regular basis.

Peter also had problems with his behavior at home. He lived with his mother, who gave birth to him when she was sixteen. He never met his father. Peter's mother could not manage his oppositional behaviors as Peter grew older. Peter stayed out past curfew and roamed the streets. He refused to help his mother around the house. She had trouble getting him up to go to school. Every morning there was a fight to get him out of bed. Peter often arrived at school late or was absent altogether. The truant officer for the school ticketed Peter's mother for not getting him to school each day and for not getting him there on time. Both Peter's teachers and his mother were frustrated.

The school strongly suggested that Peter's mother take him to a doctor to get him started on Ritalin so that he would not be suspended for the remainder of the school year. She did not want him to take Ritalin because she had heard bad things about it. She heard that it would stunt his growth for life and that it would lead to his abusing drugs and alcohol. She took him to see a counselor, who met with both of them once a week. The counselor worked with Peter's mother to develop a behavioral system whereby Peter would earn privileges for good behavior and consequences for bad behavior. Peter's behaviors did not improve. If his mother grounded him, he walked out of the house and stayed out. His mother did not know what to do and asked the counselor for help. The counselor said that his mother needed to stick to the behavioral system and not give in to Peter's behavior and that Peter would eventually improve. This did not happen.

Following are some questions for review:

1. What symptoms was Peter experiencing?
2. Does he meet the criteria for a diagnosis of any of the types of ADHD? Explain. If he does, which type?
3. Based on your current knowledge, what interventions would you suggest? Do you believe the appropriate intervention or treatment was provided?
4. Who should be included in the treatment planning and interventions?
5. What barriers might get in the way of effectively intervening?
6. What suggestions/thoughts/ideas do you have for the other members of his family?

REFERENCES

American Psychiatric Association. (1994). *Diagnostic and statistical manual of mental disorders* (4th ed.). Washington, DC: Author.

American Psychiatric Association. (2013). *Diagnostic and statistical manual of mental disorders* (5th ed.). Washington, DC: Author.

Castellanos, F. X. (2011). *ADHD in 2011: Update on research, medication treatment, and diagnostic controversies.* Retrieved from http://www.thebalancedmind.org/adhd-in -2011-update-on-research-medication-treatment-and-diagnostic-controversies?

Faraone, S. V., & Mick, E. (2010). Molecular genetics of attention deficit hyperactivity disorder. *Psychiatric Clinics of North America, 33,* 159–180.

Froehlich, T. E., Lanphear, B. P., Auinger, P., Hornung, R., Epstein, J. N., Braun, J., & Kahn, R. S. (2009). Association of tobacco and lead exposures with attention-deficit/ hyperactivity disorder. *Pediatrics, 124,* 1054–1063.

Gilliam, M., Stockman, M., Malek, M., Sharp, W., Greenstein, D., Lalonde, F., . . . Shaw, P. (2011). Developmental trajectories of the corpus callosum in attention-deficit/ hyperactivity disorder. *Biological Psychiatry, 69,* 839–846.

Gizer, I. R., Ficks, C., & Waldman, I. D. (2009). Candidate gene studies of ADHD: A meta-analytic review. *Human Genetics, 126,* 51–90.

Kieling, C., Kieling, R. R., Rohde, L. A., Frick, P. J., Moffitt, T., Nigg, J. T., . . . Castellanos, F. X. (2010). The age at onset of attention deficit hyperactivity disorder. *American Journal of Psychiatry, 167,* 14–16.

Lahey, B. B., Pelham, W. E., Loney, J., Lee, S. S., & Willcutt, E. (2005). Instability of the DSM-IV subtypes of ADHD from preschool through elementary school. *Archives of General Psychiatry, 62,* 896–902.

Millichap, J. G. (2008). Etiologic classification of attention-deficit/hyperactivity disorder. *Pediatrics, 121,* 358–365.

Millichap, J. G., & Yee, M. M. (2012). The diet factor in attention-deficit/hyperactivity disorder. *Pediatrics, 129,* 330–337.

National Institute of Mental Health. (2012). *Attention deficit hyperactivity disorder* (NIH Publication No. 12–3572). Retrieved from http://www.nimh.nih.gov/health/publica tions/attention-deficit-hyperactivity-disorder/index.shtml

Nigg, J. T., Lewis, K., Edinger, T., & Falk, M. (2012). Meta-analysis of attention-deficit/ hyperactivity disorder or attention-deficit/hyperactivity disorder symptoms, restriction diet, and synthetic food color additives. *Journal of American Academy of Child and Adolescent Psychiatry, 51,* 86–97.

Nomura, Y., Marks, D. J., & Halperin, J. M. (2010). Prenatal exposure to maternal and paternal smoking on attention deficit hyperactivity disorders symptoms and diagnosis in offspring. *Journal of Nervous and Mental Disease, 198,* 672–678.

Shaw, P., Eckstrand, K., Sharp, W., Blumenthal, J., Lerch, J. P., Greenstein, D., . . . Rapoport, J. L. (2007). Attention-deficit/hyperactivity disorder is characterized by a delay in cortical maturation. *Proceedings of the National Academy of Sciences of the United States of America, 104*(49), 19649–19654.

Shaw, P., Gornick, M., Lerch, J., Addington, A., Seal, J., Greenstein, D., . . . Rapoport, J. L. (2007). Polymorphisms of the dopamine D_4 receptor, clinical outcome, and cortical structure in attention-deficit/hyperactivity disorder. *Archives of General Psychiatry, 64*, 921–931.

Shaw, P., Malek, M., Watson, B., Sharp, W., Evans, A., & Greenstein, D. (2012). Development of cortical surface area and gyrification in attention-deficit/hyperactivity disorder. *Biological Psychiatry, 72*, 191–197.

CHAPTER 9

Treatment of Attention Deficit Hyperactivity Disorder

There are many treatments for attention deficit hyperactivity disorder (ADHD). Each person with ADHD has different needs so there is not one treatment that fits all. Treatment for ADHD can take the form of behavior therapy, family therapy, social skills training, parent skills training, psychotherapy, and medication. Education and supportive therapies are helpful for a family dealing with a child with ADHD. These treatments can help a child or adolescent experience significant improvement in symptoms and daily functioning and help caregivers of the youth understand and cope with the illness. A combination of medication and other therapies can be the most effective means of improving symptoms of ADHD and level of functioning. Even with treatment, symptoms may take time to improve. Some youth experience a decrease of symptoms with or without treatment when they enter adolescence. Others carry the symptoms into adulthood. It is also important to recognize that the side effects of untreated ADHD, such as a youth's feelings of failure, low self-esteem, depression, and social isolation, may cause more problems than the disorder itself. It is always important to promote a youth's strengths and instill a sense of competence.

PSYCHOTROPIC MEDICATIONS

Although controversial, psychotropic medication is most often the first line of treatment. The most commonly prescribed medications for treating ADHD are stimulants. Several stimulant medications have been approved by the U.S. Food and Drug Administration (FDA) for children and adolescents and found to be effective in managing attentive and impulsive symptoms in up to 80 percent of youth (National Institute of Mental Health, 2012). Imaging studies of the brain have found that neurotransmitters in the brains of persons with ADHD are reabsorbed into the neuron prematurely, keeping messages from being delivered to receptors. Stimulant medications act in the central nervous system, increasing neurotransmitters such as dopamine or norepinephrine in the brain and slowing their reabsorption so that messages can transmit effectively. This provides a calming effect and helps with reducing impulsive behavior and improving attention span.

Although stimulant medications have been found to be highly effective in treating the symptoms of ADHD, there has been and continues to be significant controversy about their use in children and adolescents. Stimulant medications are classified as schedule II drugs under the Controlled Substances Act (CSA; PL 91–513, 1970), which was enacted into law by Congress as Title II of the Comprehensive Drug Abuse Prevention and Control Act of 1970. As specified under the CSA, schedule II substances are those that meet the following criteria (CSA Schedules, 2014):

- The drug or other substance has a high potential for abuse
- The drug or other substance has currently accepted medical use in treatment in the United States or currently accepted medical use with severe restrictions
- Abuse of the drug or other substance may lead to severe psychological or physical dependence

Schedule II drugs are highly monitored by the U.S. Drug Enforcement Administration (DEA), the governmental entity with authorization to provide oversight for controlled substances. The CSA requires anyone who handles controlled substances to be registered and authorized by the DEA to ensure secure storage and maintain inventories and records of any transaction that involves controlled substances.

Only persons authorized through the DEA can prescribe stimulant medications. Due to the addictive nature of these medications, there is concern about the potential for later substance abuse. Research has not found a link to future substance abuse for children treated for ADHD with stimulants. However, stimulant medications are commonly sold on the street and abused for nonmedical reasons. A study conducted in 2011 and funded through the National Institute of Drug Abuse (NIDA) found that Ritalin was used for nonmedical reasons by 1.3 percent of eighth graders, 2.6 percent of tenth graders, and 2.6 percent of twelfth graders in the study. Adderall was abused by 1.7 percent of eighth graders, 4.6 percent of tenth graders, and 6.5 percent of twelfth graders in the study. It is also not uncommon for caregivers with addictions to take their children to the doctor to get prescriptions for these controlled substances so that they can take the medication themselves.

The long-term effects of stimulant medications are not known. There is evidence that youth experience stunted growth (in both height and weight) while taking stimulants (American Academy of Pediatrics, 2001). Some research suggests that the stunted growth resolves once the medication has been stopped, but this issue continues to be studied. Other long-term consequences of taking these medications are not yet known.

All medications have potential minor and serious side effects. Most people experience no side effects or very minimal side effects from medications including stimulants. When side effects are experienced, they usually dissipate after a few days or weeks. Only a very small percentage of people experience serious side effects from a medication. Most often, serious side effects result from a combination of the medication and another physical or mental health problem. All medications should be taken as prescribed under the supervision of a medical health professional. If any side effects are experienced, the treating physician should be notified immediately.

Serious side effects from stimulant medications, including increased blood pressure and heart rate and even sudden death, have been found in children with heart problems. Stimulants also have the potential to worsen or result in new psychiatric problems. In some persons they have been reported to cause new or worsened aggressive behavior, hostility, psychotic symptoms, and thought problems. It is always important for a treating physician to be aware of this history. Youth with a history or family history of suicide, bipolar disorder, or depression should be evaluated and monitored closely. Each medication also has the potential to result in other side effects. Common FDA-approved stimulant medications and side effects are listed in Table 9.1.

There is one FDA-approved, non-stimulant medication for treating ADHD called Strattera (atomoxetine). Strattera is nonaddictive. It provides an alternative treatment for those concerned about the effects of stimulants on youth. It has been found to cause serious side effects in a small population of those studied in clinical trials (i.e., stunted growth, suicidal thoughts and actions, heart-related problems, and serious liver damage) in addition to the more common side effects of decreased appetite, nausea or vomiting, dizziness, mood swings, and drowsiness.

It is important to watch for serious side effects and changes in behaviors for all medications. When a medication does not seem to be reducing the symptoms of ADHD, it is important to advocate for an alternative treatment. However, it is also necessary to allow medications enough time to affect symptoms. Some medications act faster than others. As always, it is important to work closely with a treating physician to determine the best treatment for a child or adolescent. Psychotropic medications have not been found to normalize behavior in youth with ADHD. Even with medication, youth continue to experience poor academic achievement and problems functioning.

PSYCHOTHERAPY

Psychotherapy can be effective in helping manage the behavioral symptoms that are experienced with ADHD. Psychotherapy is often used as a generic term referring to mental health treatment in the form of talking to a mental health provider. There are other terms commonly used to mean the same thing, such as counseling, talk therapy, or therapy. There are many approaches to psychotherapy. These approaches differ based on the individual, the individual's family, and the problem being treated. Milder symptoms of ADHD may be responsive to psychotherapy without the use of medications. Psychotherapy may also be indicated when medications are not effective.

Table 9.1.   ADHD medications

Trade name	Generic name	Dosage form	FDA-approved age	Common side effects
Adderall	Amphetamine	Tablet	3 years and older	Seizures Blurred vision
Adderall XR	Amphetamine (extended release)	Extended release	6 years and older	Headache Stomachache Trouble sleeping Decreased appetite Nervousness Dizziness
Dexedrine	Dextro-amphetamine	Capsule, (extended release)	3 years and older	Fast heartbeat Decreased appetite Tremors Headache Trouble sleeping Dizziness Stomach upset Weight loss Dry mouth
Dextrostat	Dextro-amphetamine	Tablets	3 years and older	Fast heartbeat Tremors Trouble sleeping Stomach upset Dry mouth Decreased appetite Headache Dizziness Weight loss
Concerta	Methylphenidate (long acting)	Tablet (extended release)	6 years and older	Stomach upset Dry mouth Decreased appetite Headache Dizziness Weight loss Nervousness Trouble sleeping Anxiety Irritability Increased sweating

Table 9.1. (Continued)

Trade name	Generic name	Dosage form	FDA-approved age	Common side effects
Ritalin	Methylphenidate	Tablet	6 years and older	Loss of appetite Abdominal pain Weight loss Insomnia Tachycardia
Ritalin SR	Methylphenidate (extended release)	Tablet (extended release)		
Ritalin LA	Methylphenidate (long acting)	Long acting		
Daytrana	Methylphenidate	Patch	6 years and older	Redness, small bumps, or itching where applied Poor appetite Nausea Vomiting Stomach pain Weight loss Tics Trouble sleeping Mood swings Dizziness
Metadate ER	Methylphenidate	Tablet (extended release)	6 years and older	Loss of appetite Abdominal pain Weight loss Insomnia Tachycardia Headache Nervousness Trouble sleeping Dizziness
Metadate CD	Methylphenidate	Capsule, (extended release)		
Strattera	Atomoxetine	Capsule	6 years and older	Nausea Vomiting Fatigue Decreased appetite Abdominal pain Drowsiness

Table 9.1. (Continued)

Trade name	Generic name	Dosage form	FDA-approved age	Common side effects
Vyvanse	Lisdexafeta-mine dimesylate	Capsule	6 years and older	Anxiety Decreased appetite Nausea Diarrhea Dizziness Dry mouth Trouble sleeping Upper stomach pain Vomiting Irritability
Focalin	Dexmethyl-phenidate	Capsule	6 years and older	Abdominal pain Fever Allergic reactions Nausea Decreased appetite Seizures
Focalin XR	Dexmethyl-phenidate	Extended release		

Psychotherapeutic interventions for treating ADHD commonly use techniques such as teaching caregivers parenting skills to manage problem behaviors, teaching youth social skills to manage impulsive or aggressive behaviors and to interact in more socially appropriate ways, or using family therapies aimed at addressing issues across the family system that contribute to problem behavior. Many of the evidence-based practices/treatments incorporate one or all of these types of interventions.

Defiant Teen and Defiant Children

Defiant Teen and Defiant Children, developed by Russell A. Barkley (2006), are examples of two skills training curricula that integrate evidence-based practices for managing youth with ADHD. Barkley developed the curricula based on research that supports each procedure utilized throughout the manual. The program provides a structured methodology for training parents to manage problem behavior in children and adolescents. The skills are meant to be taught sequentially because each new skill is built on previous skills. These skills training curricula provide family training in parental management skills, understanding the underlying correlates of social learning of childhood defiant behavior, and use of positive attention as a means to improve parental management skills and competence in dealing with behavior problems, particularly noncompliant or defiant behavior. Guidelines for therapists in conducting each step of the program, assessment materials, and handouts are included.

The child curriculum consists of ten self-contained training units and the adolescent version contains eighteen units. The units can be incorporated into family therapy or parent counseling and can be offered individually or in a group format. Each session follows a standardized pattern. The overarching goal of the curricula is to improve family harmony by meeting the following objectives:

- To increase parental knowledge of the causes of childhood defiant behavior;
- To improve caregiver use of positive attention;
- To teach caregivers to provide clear guidance, rules, and instruction to their children;
- To teach caregivers to provide swift, fair, and just discipline for inappropriate behavior.

The first half of both curricula consists of teaching caregivers a series of behavior management tactics to employ with their child. The curricula follow the same core components for managing challenging youth behavior (see Table 9.2). Both curricula include the Skills Development and Enhancement Model, which focuses on teaching parents about causes of problem behaviors and developing specific parenting skills. The adolescent version includes Graduated Problem-Solving and Communication Training, which teaches parents and adolescents methods of proper problem solving and communication skills for negotiating through conflict.

Defiant Teen and Defiant Children are examples of curricula based on evidence-based practices, but they are not considered evidence-based treatments. Providers are not required to participate in any training by the developer. The following subsections will provide a few examples of evidence-based treatments for ADHD.

Challenging Horizons Program

The Challenging Horizons Program (CHP) is an empirically supported, school-based treatment program developed for students from ages six through

Table 9.2. Core components of Defiant Child and Defiant Teen curricula

Skills Development and Enhancement Model
- Impose immediate positive or negative consequences in response to the child's behavior;
- Impose consequences that are specific to the behavior being addressed;
- Make all consequences predictable, contingent, and discriminate;
- Establish incentive programs for rewarding the appropriate alternative behavior before punishing negative behaviors;
- Make consequences consistent across settings, over time, and between caregivers;
- Anticipate problematic behaviors and develop methods that will reduce the probability of those problems developing;
- Recognize and modify unreasonable beliefs, thoughts, and expectations that caregivers have about their child;
- Recognize that family interactions are reciprocal and change the parent's unilateral view that either they caused the problem or the problem is the teen's fault.

Graduated Problem-Solving and Communication Training
- Gradually allow the youth increased developmentally appropriate independence;
- Distinguish behaviors and consequences that are negotiable from those that are nonnegotiable;
- Involve adolescents in problem solving for negotiable issues;
- Maintain good communication between caregivers and youth;
- Develop realistic expectations of family hierarchy.

seventeen who are experiencing ADHD (Evans, Langberg, Raggi, Allen, & Buvinger, 2005; Langberg et al., 2006). This program combines behavioral and cognitive interventions with supportive counseling. It targets social impairment, family conflict, and academic problems. The goals of CHP are to improve academic achievement, confidence, motivation, attendance, and behaviors. Providers of CHP must participate in fifteen hours of off-site training and ongoing supervision; schools providing CHP must be accredited annually. Accredited sites are required to adhere to a set of core components:

- Low student to staff ratio;
- An environment that is safe and engaging and provides social reinforcement, tangible rewards, and clear and consistently enforced rules;
- Training in enabling skills, such as organization;
- Training in specific educational skills, such as math and reading;
- Emphasis on improving social skills;
- Emphasis on goal setting and improving self-regulation of behavior;
- Parental involvement through group parent training and weekly reports;

- Participation in continuous quality improvement assisted by manuals, preservice training, on-site supervision and feedback using fidelity forms, and empirical evaluation of CHP activities.

Two versions of CHP have been developed, evaluated, and found to be effective for managing symptoms and behaviors associated with ADHD. In the after-school model, counselors and trained providers meet with groups of five to twenty students with ADHD two to three times a week. A ratio of one staff person for every two to three group members is required to ensure that students receive individual help and attention. During the group sessions, students receive training in organizational skills, problem-solving skills, study skills, assignment tracking, note taking, pro-social skills, and self-monitoring of behaviors. Counselors maintain regular contact with teachers and caregivers to monitor progress. The second version of CHP, the consulting model, is provided by school staff such as teachers or counselors trained in CHP. Individual sessions are conducted with students during the school day and focus on the same goals as the after-school version.

Parenting with Love and Limits

Parenting with Love and Limits (PLL; Sells, 1998) is a widely used evidence-based practice that combines group and family therapies. It was developed for treating youth from ages ten through eighteen with severe emotional and behavioral problems, including ADHD. Families participate in six 1- to 2-hour didactic group sessions with as many as six other families. Sessions are led by two trained therapists. Each session focuses on a specific topic aimed at teaching caregivers new information and skills designed to reestablish their parental authority through consistent limits and a loving relationship. During the first hour, parents and youth meet together. They split into separate groups during the second hour. Table 9.3 shows the topics and goals of each session.

Families also participate in individual family therapy sessions. The number of family therapy sessions in which a family participates depends on the level of family problems. It can range from three sessions for families whose children have moderate behavioral problems to as many as twenty sessions for families whose child exhibits more severe behavioral problems. During and between therapy sessions, parents and youth practice skills to enhance what they have learned.

Table 9.3. Session agenda for Parenting with Love and Limits

Weekly topic	Goals of session
Week 1: Understanding why your teen misbehaves	To teach caregivers the reasons why teens act out and to prevent teens from regaining control.
Week 2: Button pushing	To teach youth and caregivers how and why button pushing creates family conflict and how to identify buttons that escalate fights.
Week 3: Why traditional behavioral contracts fail and the art of negotiation	To teach families how to negotiate and design their own rewards.
Week 4: Writing new contracts and the use of emotional warm-ups	To teach parents how to develop behavioral contracts and how to present the contracts to their children. To teach youth how to reduce conflict and enhance relationships.
Week 5: Pulling it all together	To teach parents how to use creative consequences to stop problem behaviors and how to create a Positive Teen Report Certificate and use it to catch children acting positively.
Week 6: Restoring lost nurturance and tenderness (if needed)	To educate families on reactive attachment and to teach them how the fine line between love and dislike works and why there is a current lack of nurturance.
Week 7 and beyond: Ongoing coaching (if needed)	To reduce problems at home and school and with the law.

Agencies/programs that provide PLL must be licensed annually. The cost for annual licensing is approximately $1,500 per family served plus travel expenses. Providers receive a five-day training, regular telephone consultation, annual on-site consultation, and videotaped therapist supervision.

CASE STUDIES

Eric

Eric is the ten-year-old who was removed from his mother's care by Child Protective Services for physical abuse and placed with his grandmother. Eric had no contact with his father or his father's family. He was allowed to see his mother as long as his grandmother was present.

In school, Eric was antsy and could not remain seated. He refused to do his schoolwork and did not get along with the other children. He did not have any friends and did not participate in any activities with other kids. By the age of ten he had been kicked out of two elementary schools, the last one for stabbing another student with a pencil.

When Eric moved in with his grandmother, she took him to a community mental health center. She reported that he had tried to hang himself twice and was all over the place. Eric received medication for ADHD and depression and attended counseling once a week. His grandmother met with the therapist at the end of every appointment to give an update on his week. Each week for nearly three years, Eric's grandmother reported that he continued to be out of control and to experience episodes. When his counselor tried to talk with Eric about his mother and his suicide attempts, all he would say is that he did not remember. When asked why he continued to have episodes at home, he would say something negative about himself.

Eric's counselor moved out of the area and Eric met with a new counselor. After looking through his records, the new counselor decided that she needed more information from other sources. She met with Eric's teachers and principal. He had been transferred to this school after being expelled from another school. His teachers reported that Eric's behavior had improved considerably; they felt that the improvement was due to the expectation that he could behave appropriately. They chose not to listen to the problems he had experienced at past schools. They all felt that he was very bright and reported that he was doing very well academically, going from failing to making the honor roll.

After meeting with Eric's teachers and principal, Eric's counselor scheduled a meeting at his grandmother's house and requested that his mother attend. The counselor noticed that Eric's behavior with his grandmother was very erratic, and that his grandmother seemed to say things that set him off. He acted lovingly and appropriately with his mother. The counselor felt that it would be important for the family to have in-home services and to include his mother in the treatment as well.

The family was referred into wraparound and in-home skills training services. The wraparound team consisted of Eric, his grandmother, his mother, his English teacher, and his Child Protective Services case worker. In wraparound meetings, Eric's mother reported that she wanted Eric to eventually move back with her. The grandmother became very angry at this idea and refused to attend any more wraparound meetings or skills training sessions. The rest of the team continued to meet and devised a wraparound plan that included increasing contact between Eric and his mother and monitoring how things went. When he was with his mother, Eric behaved very well. The skills trainer noted that Eric's mother was working very hard and incorporating skills that she had learned in sessions. Eric ended up returning to live with his mother. He was taken off all medications and continued to do well in school, to make friends, and to participate in pro-social activities. After a year, Child Protective Services closed his case.

Peter

Peter is the twelve-year-old seventh grader who was failing all of his classes and tested below his grade level on standardized tests. He was the class clown who made jokes and did things to make classmates laugh. He teachers were unable to redirect him, and he became oppositional. He was sent to the office for his behaviors and for disturbing class regularly.

Peter also had problems with his behavior at home. He lived with his mother, who gave birth to him when she was sixteen. Peter's mother could not control his behaviors. He broke curfew regularly and roamed the streets. He refused to help his mother around the house. She had trouble getting him up to go to school. His mother was ticketed for not getting him to school each day and for not getting him there on time.

The school strongly suggested that Peter's mother take him to a doctor to get him started on Ritalin so that he would not be suspended for the remainder of the school year. His mother did not want him to take Ritalin because she had heard bad things about it. Instead, she took him to see a counselor who met with both of them once a week. The counselor worked with his mother to develop a behavioral system whereby Peter would earn privileges for good behavior and consequences for bad behavior. The behavioral plan was ineffective in managing Peter's behaviors. Finally, his mother decided to take him to see a psychiatrist, who prescribed Adderall. The Adderall helped Peter focus at school and stop squirming around. He continued to get in trouble at home and school.

Consider the following questions:

1. What do these real life scenarios have in common?
2. What are the differences?
3. After learning what happened to each of the youths, do you have any different thoughts on how you would have handled the situation if you were the families' social worker?

REFERENCES

American Academy of Pediatrics. (2001). Clinical practice guideline: Treatment of the school-aged child with attention deficit/hyperactivity disorder. *Pediatrics, 108,* 1033–1044.

Barkley, R. A. (2006). *Attention-deficit/hyperactivity disorder: A handbook for diagnosis and treatment* (3rd ed.). New York: Guilford Press.

Controlled Substances Act of 1970, Pub. L. No. 91–513 § 84 Stat. 1242 (1970).

CSA Schedules. (2014). Retrieved from http://www.drugs.com/csa-schedule.html

Evans, S. W., Langberg, J., Raggi, V., Allen, J., & Buvinger, E. (2005). Development of a school-based treatment program for middle school youth with ADHD. *Journal of Attention Disorders, 9,* 343–353.

Langberg, J., Smith, B. H., Bogle, K. E., Schmidt, J. D., Cole, W. R., & Pender, C. A. (2006). A pilot evaluation of small group Challenging Horizons Program (CHP): A randomized trial. *Journal of Applied School Psychology, 23,* 31–58.

National Institute of Mental Health. (2012). *Attention deficit hyperactivity disorder* (NIH Publication No. 12–3572). Retrieved from http://www.nimh.nih.gov/health/publica tions/attention-deficit-hyperactivity-disorder/index.shtml

Sells, S. P. (1998). *Treating the tough adolescent: A step-by-step, family-based guide.* New York: Guilford Press.

CHAPTER 10

Conduct Disorder and Oppositional Defiant Disorder

BECAUSE OF THEIR PREVALENCE and the disruption that they cause, not only to children's lives, but also to the lives of those around them, two of the most problematic mental health disorders of childhood and adolescence are oppositional defiant disorder (ODD) and conduct disorder (CD). Youth who develop CD or ODD often have experienced physical abuse, sexual abuse, neglect, poverty, and/or family dysfunction; therefore, youth in the juvenile justice and child welfare systems are highly susceptible to developing one of these disorders (Farmer, Compton, Burns, & Robertson, 2002).

Both disorders are often referred to as *externalizing disorders* in that their symptoms are characterized by acting out behaviors and defiance of authority. Youth with these disorders are the youth who are moved from foster home to foster home, who end up in residential treatment, or who come in contact with the juvenile justice system due to the difficulty and challenges their behaviors pose. Left untreated, these externalizing disorders can develop into chronic delinquency that will disrupt positive development and can follow the youth into adulthood (Farmer et al., 2002; Hill, Coie, Lochman, & Greenberg, 2004). The result could be criminal activity, unemployment, substance abuse, ineffective parenting, and relationship problems. The children of these youth are then at risk of becoming the next generation in the juvenile justice, mental health, and child welfare systems. If we identify and treat these problems, we are not only improving the lives of these youth, but we are helping to stop a generational cycle of abuse and neglect, criminal activity, or other problems. The first step in this process is identifying and understanding the problem.

OPPOSITIONAL DEFIANT DISORDER

Oppositional defiant disorder is a less severe behavioral disorder than conduct disorder; however, it is still disruptive to a youth's functioning and development and very challenging to those around him or her. Youth with ODD are characterized by inflexibility, negative mood, and hostility (American Psychiatric Association, 2013). Their overall view of life tends to be negative. They focus on the negative aspects of themselves, others, and situations rather finding the positive aspects. These youth often have poor problem-solving and coping skills and thus respond to the environment and others in negative ways. Youth experiencing symptoms of ODD can be highly irritable and respond to even small problems or things that bother them with intense anger. Their intense anger and hostile response are often used to control others. One consequence of this way of responding is poor relationships with peers, teachers, and family.

Signs of ODD are usually evident before the age of eight (American Psychiatric Association, 2013). A child with ODD is the child who *consistently* refuses to comply with requests from authority figures or does not comply within a reasonable amount of time or to the degree expected. For example, when a caregiver requests the child to do something, such as clean his or her bedroom, the child generally refuses to comply and responds by screaming and yelling things such as "this is unfair; I hate you." The child may finally go to his or her room, but rather than cleaning it as expected, he or she will push all the dirty clothes under the bed instead of putting them in the dirty clothes hamper. This is the child who is prone to throwing temper tantrums or even possibly making physical threats in order to get his or her way. This is not the child who occasionally does not want to clean his or her room. This is the child whose response to requests is extreme for the situation. When confronted with a task with which he or she is struggling or that he or she perceives as too difficult, the child tends to give up and move on to another activity. If someone pushes him or her to complete the task, for example, to finish homework, he or she will respond by screaming and yelling, hitting objects, or engaging in other extreme behavioral responses rather than working through the problem.

These behaviors may sound like normal youth behavior. However, for a diagnosis of ODD, the behaviors must be occurring at a level that is more intense or frequent than would be expected for a youth at the same developmental stage (American Psychiatric Association, 2013). To the persons around the youth, everything seems to be spiraling out of control. The problems rise to a level that is seriously affecting the youth's functioning, relationships, or success in school and causing significant stress for caregivers.

DIAGNOSING OPPOSITIONAL DEFIANT DISORDER

The *Diagnostic and Statistical Manual of Mental Disorders* (*DSM*) spells out the criteria for a diagnosis. As specified in the *DSM*, in order to be diagnosed with ODD, a youth must be younger than eighteen and exhibit four or more of the following behaviors for at least six months:

- Often loses temper
- Often argues with adults
- Often actively defies or refuses to comply with adults' requests or rules
- Often deliberately annoys people
- Often blames others for his or her mistakes or misbehavior
- Is often touchy or easily annoyed by others
- Is often angry and resentful
- Is often spiteful or vindictive

The changes from the *DSM-IV* (American Psychiatric Association, 1994) to the *DSM-5* (American Psychiatric Association, 2013) were minor for ODD. The main change in the *DSM-5* is a new emphasis on a persistent pattern of angry and irritable mood along with vindictive behavior (Dickstein, 2010). The behaviors identified in the *DSM-5* as characteristic of ODD are divided into three symptom clusters: angry/irritable, touchy/easily annoyed by others, and angry/resentful. However, the number (four) and duration of symptoms required for an ODD diagnosis have not changed. The intensity is specified based on age, with the requirement that those younger than five experience symptoms almost every day and those who are five or older experience symptoms at least once a week.

There are no blood tests, brain scans, or other biological tests that can be conducted to diagnose ODD. In order to make the diagnosis, a mental health professional must interview a youth face to face and obtain reliable information from others such as a caregiver, teacher, or other person involved with the youth. The evaluation should explore the youth's development, the family history of mental health and substance abuse problems, and the youth's functioning at school and home and in the community. The mental health professional should explore whether the youth may have another problem that is the true explanation for the behavior. It is not uncommon for depressed youth, particularly males, to express their depression in a way that looks like ODD. It is also likely that there is a coexisting issue such as attention deficit hyperactivity disorder (ADHD) or a learning disability that confounds the problem. It is essential for a correct diagnosis or diagnoses to be made. This is not possible without an in-depth evaluation. If the correct problem or a coexisting problem is not identified, we will waste our effort and not see improvement with the youth. It is important not to blame the youth or the caregiver because treatment may not have been directed at the right problem. Effective treatment is impossible without targeting the correct problem or coexisting conditions.

CONDUCT DISORDER

Oppositional defiant disorder is often seen as a precursor to conduct disorder (CD) and/or substance abuse. Approximately a third of youth with ODD go on to develop CD (Dickstein, 2010). The good news is that approximately two-thirds of youth do not develop CD and may simply grow out of the problem behaviors. Children and teens with CD are thought of by the general public as juvenile delinquents rather than as youth with a mental illness. As previously stated, CD is a more serious and disruptive behavioral disorder than ODD. Youth with CD exhibit patterns of violating the rights of others and/or violating social rules (American Psychiatric Association, 2013). Often a lack of empathy or remorse accompanies these behaviors. If asked why they do certain things, youth with CD will often respond that they were bored. They lack the ability to read social cues. For instance, a happenstance eye glance in their direction may be misinterpreted as confrontational and trigger a strong reaction, such as threatening behavior. Youth with CD are more likely to abuse illegal substances and engage in risk-taking behavior. These youth typically have significant juvenile justice involvement. Violations of rules and of other people, lack of empathy or remorse, and inability to read social cues result in significant levels of impairment in daily functioning, particularly in relationship problems.

DIAGNOSING CONDUCT DISORDER

As with ODD, CD is diagnosed through a face-to-face diagnostic interview with a mental health professional and not with a blood test or brain scan. To receive a diagnosis of CD, a person must be younger than eighteen and have exhibited three or more behaviors in the past twelve months (at least one in the past six months) that involved aggression against people or animals, serious violation of rules, destruction of property, and/or deceitfulness or theft. The *DSM-V* (American Psychiatric Association, 2013) identifies behaviors under each of these four categories:

1. Aggression against people and animals
    a. Often bullies, threatens, or intimidates others;
    b. Often initiates physical fights;
    c. Has used a weapon that can cause serious physical harm to others;
    d. Has been physically cruel to people;
    e. Has been physically cruel to animals;
    f. Has stolen while confronting a victim (e.g., mugging, purse snatching, extortion, or armed robbery);
    g. Has forced someone into sexual activity.
2. Destruction of property
    a. Has deliberately engaged in fire setting with the intention of causing serious damage;
    b. Has deliberately destroyed others' property (other than by fire setting).

3. Deceitfulness or theft
   a. Has broken into someone else's house, building, or car;
   b. Often lies to obtain goods or favors or to avoid obligations (i.e., cons others);
   c. Has stolen items of nontrivial value without confronting a victim (e.g., shoplifting, but without breaking and entering or forgery).

4. Serious violations of rules
   a. Often stays out at night despite parental prohibitions, beginning before age thirteen;
   b. Has run away from home overnight at least twice while living in parental or parental surrogate home (or once without returning for a lengthy period);
   c. Is often truant from school, beginning before age thirteen.

The only significant change in diagnosing CD from the *DSM-IV* to the *DSM-5* is the addition of the specifier *with or without callous and unemotional traits*. For the specifier with callous and unemotional traits, two or more of the following characteristics should be persistently evident for at least twelve months and in more than one setting or relationship (American Psychiatric Association, 2013):

- *Lack of remorse or guilt*: Does not feel bad or guilty when he or she does something wrong (except if expressing remorse when caught and/ or facing punishment).
- *Callousness and lack of empathy*: Disregards and is unconcerned about the feelings of others.
- *Lack of concern about performance*: Does not show concern about poor/ problematic performance at school or work or in other important activities.
- *Shallow or deficient affect*: Does not express feelings or show emotions to others except in ways that seem shallow or superficial (e.g., emotions are not consistent with actions; can turn emotions on or off quickly) or when they are used for gain (e.g., to manipulate or intimidate others).

As with ADHD, the *DSM-5* encourages the clinician to ensure the accuracy of information obtained by collecting information from multiple sources (e.g., caregivers, teachers, and grandparents) before making the diagnosis of conduct disorder with callous and unemotional traits.

Although people may continue to carry a diagnosis of conduct disorder past the age of eighteen, even if they do not fully meet the criteria, most often the diagnosis will change to antisocial personality disorder. Conduct disorder and antisocial personality disorder share many similarities (American Psychiatric Association, 2013). Antisocial personality disorder is a chronic disorder. Someone with the disorder perceives situations and relates to others in an abnormal, destructive manner. These are the adults who have been sent to prison for committing severe acts of violence and who lack remorse for their actions. All youth with CD do not go on to have antisocial disorder as adults; however, evidence suggests that they are at a high risk because personality disorders are thought to have roots in childhood delinquency (Farmer et al., 2002; Hill et al., 2004). Children whose behaviors early on involve violence and aggression against others are at the highest risk for antisocial personality disorder. As children age, their behaviors may become more aggressive and violent and occur more frequently. The differences between those who do and those who do not go on to exhibit criminal activity as adults are the level and type of intervention they receive as youth and the age at which they receive it.

CAUSES AND CORRELATES OF OPPOSITIONAL DEFIANT DISORDER AND CONDUCT DISORDER

Many risk factors contribute to the development of ODD or CD. Youth who have experienced child abuse or neglect or who have caregivers with similar oppositional or criminal traits and characteristics have a higher risk of developing one of these disorders. No single factor results in the disorders; rather it is the culmination of risk factors that come together (Henggeler, Schoenwald, Rowland, & Cunningham, 2002). These factors include caregiver, youth, community, and peer group characteristics.

Caregiver Characteristics

Many caregiver characteristics place youth at risk of developing ODD or CD (Dickstein, 2010; Fergusson, Lynskey, & Horwood, 1993; Frick et al., 1992). Caregivers experiencing high levels of stress with low educational levels, lack of social support, and inability to cope with or manage the stress often respond by lashing out at others around them or retreating from others. Studies have found a strong correlation between youth problem behaviors and maternal depression, stress, or marital discord (Christensen, Phillips, Glasgow, & Johnson, 1983; Dumas, Gibson, & Albin, 1989; Fergusson et al., 1993; Nigg & Hinshaw, 1998). When a mother is experiencing depression, she is more likely to be neglectful of her children due to a lack of interest or ability to parent. Children from neglectful households are characterized by poorer adjustment than those from other types of households. They are more likely to use drugs and alcohol and participate in delinquent behavior.

Research has also found a strong association between parental and child externalizing disorders suggesting a familial transmission. Specifically, caregivers who lack concern for societal rules and lack empathy have a high probability of having children who develop similar temperamental characteristics. It is not unknown for parents to take a child with negative acting out behavior to see a mental health professional and to report difficulty in understanding where their children's behavior comes from right after yelling at the check-in staff about having what they perceived was a long wait to see the counselor.

Caregivers (usually paternal) with antisocial disorder are more likely to have children who develop ODD or CD than other caregivers. Antisocial personality disorder is similar to CD in that people with the disorder violate societal rules and the rights of others. They perceive situations abnormally and thus behave in an abnormal manner, such as with violence. Adults with antisocial personality disorder likely had CD as youth.

Another of the major causes of noncompliance, defiance, and social aggression is poor, ineffective, inconsistent, and indiscriminant child or teen management by parents, often combined with unusually harsh or extreme disciplinary methods and poor monitoring of teen activities (Henggeler, Schoenwald, Borduin, Rowland, & Cunningham, 1998; Henggeler et al., 2002). Parents with an authoritarian parenting style are directive and controlling and exhibit low levels of comfort and warmth to their children. Their punishment style tends to be severe and often physically abusive. This style of parenting has been linked to aggression, poor self-confidence, internalized distress, and social withdrawal in children. Children living in authoritarian households are not allowed to experience the natural consequences of their behaviors.

On the other extreme is the permissive style of parenting. Permissive parents can be very loving; some want to be their child's friend rather than parent. However, they do not provide or maybe cannot provide structure or discipline and thus they allow their children to exhibit impulsive or other behaviors without any consequence. Children living in households with a permissive form of parenting may exhibit impulsive, aggressive behavior and a lack of social responsibility.

Youth Characteristics

Children are all born with unique temperaments that affect how they interact and respond to the world. Temperament is different from personality in that temperament is a core characteristic. It is consistent across time. Personality is a combination of life experiences and core characteristics. The temperament of youth who develop ODD or CD tends to be negative and inflexible. This temperament results in their experiencing problems in adapting to different situations. They exhibit poor social skills and/or problem-solving skills. They often have difficulty managing their own behavior, resulting in heightened reactions that are more extreme than would be expected for the situation. These characteristics can exacerbate problems in relationships between the child and caregivers, peers, and teachers. People often find themselves frustrated with the child's behavior and react to it in ways that are not consistent with their normal behavior. Children or teens having certain temperaments and cognitive characteristics are more prone to exhibit coercive-aggressive behavior and noncompliance than other teens or children.

Peer and Community Characteristics

The larger contextual events surrounding a family, both internal and external, create or contribute to increased risk of a youth developing ODD or CD. A vast amount of research exists on the influence of peer groups on youth behavior (Henggeler et al., 1998, 2002). A child or teen who hangs out with friends who abuse substances and participate in criminal and delinquent behavior is more likely to interact with these same behaviors than a youth who has friends who participate in pro-social activities. Understandably, caregivers of youth who participate in pro-social activities will not want their children to be involved with youth known to be delinquent for fear that they will negatively influence their child. This makes it more difficult for youth with a history of delinquency to change to a peer group that would be a positive influence.

The community surrounding a youth also has a great influence on development of problem behaviors. Communities that lack opportunities for youth to participate in pro-social activities such as organized sports or boy or girl scouts have also been linked to youth problem behavior due to boredom. Youth who live in communities with high levels of crime and violence are at an increased risk of becoming involved in criminal and violent activity.

Youth spend much of their time in a school setting. School settings can have a significant influence on youth behavior. Schools with rigid rules and negative teacher-student interactions can have a negative effect on youth behavior. Many youth with a behavior disorder also have a learning disability. Placement in an appropriate educational setting with teachers who are knowledgeable and skilled, not only in dealing with the learning disability, but also in managing behavioral problems in the classroom, is imperative. It can take a certain temperament to work with youths with conduct disorder.

THE BRAIN AND CONDUCT DISORDER

Findings of research on abnormalities in the brains of youth with CD could change the way we think about its development. The emerging evidence suggests that antisocial and aggressive behavior is attributable to these abnormalities rather than to peer pressure (Passamonti et al., 2010; Sterzer, Stadler, Poustka, & Kleinschmidt, 2007). Evidence suggests that youth with CD have abnormalities in brain structures and functioning that contribute to its onset and associated behaviors (Fairchild et al., 2011; Passamonti et al., 2010; van Goozen & Fairchild, 2006; van Goozen, Fairchild, Snoek, & Harold, 2007). More recent studies are finding that adolescents with CD experience abnormal neural activity when processing the facial expressions of others (Fairchild, van Goozen, Calder, Stollery, & Goodyer, 2009). Impairment to the frontal lobe results in poor impulse control, difficulty learning from past experiences, and difficulty planning for the future (Fairchild, van Goozen, Stollery, et al., 2009). Decreased serotonin and cortisol levels and decreased grey matter in the amygdala have also been found in youth with CD. These differences may explain their lack of fear, decreased ability to control aggressive and impulsive behaviors, and inability to recognize emotional reactions of others. When youth are unable to understand others' reactions, particularly distress, they are unable to exhibit empathy. Studies have found that youth who have callous and unemotional traits have less activity in their amygdala than other youth with CD and are those exhibiting lack of empathy for others (Marsh et al., 2008).

COMORBIDITY WITH OTHER DISORDERS

The most common disorder found to be comorbid (or commonly occurring together) with both ODD and CD is ADHD (American Psychiatric Association, 2013; National Institute of Mental Health, 2012). It is believed that nearly 50 percent of youth with ODD also have ADHD and as many as 30 percent of boys and 55 percent of girls with CD also experience ADHD (National Institute of Mental Health, 2012). Depression has also been found to be linked to both ODD and CD. Some youth experiencing depression may exhibit symptoms of ODD or CD and have the problem with depression undiagnosed. Youth with a dual diagnosis of CD and ADHD have been found to be more aggressive than youth with CD alone. Conduct disorder is often found to be comorbid with several other mental health, substance use/abuse, and learning disorders (National Institute of Mental Health, 2012). Youth with CD have been found to begin use/abuse of alcohol and drugs at an earlier age than other youth and are more likely to use more types of substances. The most common learning disability found to be comorbid with CD is language impairments, affecting as many as 25 percent of youth with CD.

IMPLICATIONS FOR FOSTER YOUTH

As we know, youth in the child welfare system are at a higher risk than other children of having or developing CD or ODD due to the high correlation of these disorders with physical abuse, neglect, poverty, and family dysfunction. Think about the characteristics of caregivers who come in contact with the child welfare system. Many possess characteristics correlated with a child or teen developing ODD or CD. Caregivers coming in contact with the child welfare system are most likely the ones experiencing high levels of stress and having poor coping skills and/or a mental health problem such as major depression or bipolar disorder.

Although youth in the foster care system do possess many of the risk factors associated with ODD and CD, it is for this very reason that we must be careful in assessing these disorders. We should not jump to the conclusion that a youth who is acting out has one of these disorders and ignore other plausible causes of this behavior. There are many reasons for acting out behavior. The youth may be responding to the stress of being removed from home, siblings, school, and friends and placed in an unfamiliar setting with strangers. It is understandable that a child or teenager, even one who normally can cope with stress, would act out in response to such an extreme change in his or her life. It is important to remember that different youth will respond in different ways based on their own characteristics, such as temperament, stress management skills, and coping skills. Given time and positive support, these acting out behaviors may cease. At the same time, if the youth is not provided support and time to deal with what is happening to him or her, the behaviors may persist even to the point of developing into one of these externalizing disorders.

Sometimes youth experiencing other mental health disorders may exhibit acting out behaviors that are masking the true mental health problem. This can be particularly true for males with depression. Females tend to exhibit the symptoms we picture when thinking about depression. Males on the other hand sometimes exhibit anger and acting out behavior in response to depression. It is also important to understand that ODD and CD are often comorbid with other mental health problems. Common mental health problems that can coexist with ODD or CD are depression, anxiety, ADHD, learning disabilities, or one or more other problems.

It is important for social workers to ensure that all children or teenagers entering child welfare receive a trauma-informed comprehensive psycho-social, emotional, behavioral, educational, and biological assessment in order to provide them with the best care possible. Acting out behaviors attract attention because of the irritation they cause case workers, service providers, and foster parents. If our response to the youth's behavior is to keep moving him or her from foster home to foster home or into residential placement, the youth has been set up for failure. If we do not identify the correct problem(s), chances are that any interventions provided will not be successful. A child presenting with ODD symptoms should have a comprehensive evaluation. It is important to look for other disorders that may be present, such as ADHD, learning disabilities, mood disorders (depression, or bipolar disorder), and anxiety disorders. It may be difficult to improve the symptoms of ODD without treating the coexisting disorder.

CASE STUDIES

Following are some case studies of youth experiencing behavioral problems. To protect their privacy, we will not use their real names. As you read each story, think about the symptoms being exhibited and which disorder you believe the youth is experiencing. All of these youths were diagnosed with either ODD or CD. They each received a different form of intervention, and their lives took completely different paths. Their case studies will be continued in chapter 11.

Tim

Tim is a thirteen-year-old boy. He lives with his mother and eleven-year-old sister in a public housing apartment complex. His father died when he was seven. Tim's mother, Jean, has an intellectual disability with an IQ under 90. He and his sister both have normal IQs. The family survives on Jean's social security check and social security checks Tim and his sister receive due to the death of their father.

Jean did well with raising her children when they were young. She ensured that they had clean clothes, ample food, and safe housing and that they went to school every day. She belonged to a church that provided her with support. As Tim grew older, he stopped listening to his mother. He told her that she was stupid and that he did not have to do what she said. He tormented his sister both verbally and physically. He stayed out past his curfew and hung out with friends. His first run-in with the juvenile justice system came when he and his friends were caught breaking into the school and destroying property. His mother did not know what to do to control his behavior. His second encounter with the juvenile justice system occurred when a young girl in the neighborhood reported that he had been sexually abusing her. Tim was adjudicated and mandated to attend outpatient sex offender treatment. While he was completing his treatment, it was reported that he was abusing a neighborhood boy. The judge ordered him into an inpatient sex offender treatment program. He received intensive individual and group therapy for the year he remained in the program. He was then discharged to return home.

Consider the following questions:

1. What symptoms was Tim experiencing?

2. Based on the information provided, does he meet the criteria for either of the diagnoses? Explain. If he does, which one?

3. Based on your current knowledge, what interventions would you suggest? Do you believe that he received the appropriate intervention or treatment?

4. Who should be included in Tim's treatment planning and interventions?

5. What barriers might get in the way of effectively intervening with Tim?

6. What suggestions/thoughts/ideas do you have for the other members of Tim's family?

Tracy

Tracy is an eight-year-old girl. She had always exhibited difficult behavior such as throwing a tantrum when she did not get her way, but her negative and acting out behavior became increasingly unbearable. She was getting in trouble at school more frequently. She talked back to her teachers and sometimes refused to do her work. Many of the children in her classroom did not like her because she made fun of them or tried to get them in trouble by telling the teacher that they had started a fight with her. When a teacher confronted her about lying, Tracy started yelling and said that she did not lie. She walked out of her classroom and down the hall. The teacher caught up with her and they walked together to the principal's office. She received a three-day in-school suspension. At home she was mean to her little brother. Often, when her mother asked her to put her school books and toys in her room or to do some other chore, Tracy would reply, "I will do it when my favorite show is over." If her mother pressed her, she would sometimes comply; however, more often, she would scream and yell and run to her room and slam the door. Tracy's mother was at her wits' end and took her to see a counselor.

Write your answers to the following questions:

1. What symptoms was Tracy experiencing?

2. Does she meet the criteria for either CD or ODD? Explain. If she does, which one?

3. Based on your current knowledge, what interventions would you suggest? Do you believe that she received the appropriate intervention or treatment?

4. Who should be included in Tracy's treatment planning and interventions?

5. What barriers might get in the way of effectively intervening with Tracy?

6. What suggestions/thoughts/ideas do you have for the other members of her family?

James

James is a seventeen-year-old living with both his parents in a middle class neighborhood. When his father was not home, James talked back and cursed at his mother, refused to follow her rules, and threatened to hurt her. His father had more control over James's behavior. He was a large man with an explosive anger that at times became physical. James was afraid of his father. James's father worked a night shift and was not home much when James was home. James walked out of the house at any time of the night he chose and hung out with friends. They drank alcohol, smoked marijuana, and huffed glue. At school he was a bully. He was suspended and placed in an alternative school for beating up other students, skipping school, and defying his teachers. One evening, his mother tried to stop him from leaving the house. James beat her severely. Her face was bloody and so swollen that it was unrecognizable. When her husband returned home from work, he found her on the kitchen floor and called 911. James was not at home. His mother was taken to the hospital with broken ribs and bruises that covered her body. The police located James and took him to the juvenile detention center. When questioned about the incident, he at first lied and said that he did not beat up his mother. When he finally admitted to it, he said that it was his mother's fault for never shutting up.

James spent three months in juvenile detention. He was discharged to return home with an ankle monitor and strict instructions from the judge that he would be sent to a more restrictive lockup facility until he turned twenty-one if he did not comply with his probation or had any more incidences of trouble.

Think about the following questions:

1. What symptoms was James experiencing?

2. Does he meet the criteria for CD or ODD? Explain. If he does, which one?

3. Based on your current knowledge, what interventions would you suggest? Do you believe that the appropriate intervention or treatment was provided?

4. Who should be included in the treatment planning and interventions?

5. What barriers might get in the way of effectively intervening?

6. What suggestions/thoughts/ideas do you have for the other members of James's family?

Dale

Dale is a sixteen-year-old who has been in and out of the juvenile justice system since the age of thirteen for causing bodily harm to others, theft, and use of illegal drugs. He is failing in school. He spent several months in alternative school. He was placed in residential care for a year. As is common, the residential care center was located hundreds of miles from his home and his mother. While he was in care, his mother had little participation in treatment other than a monthly meeting with the social worker to discuss his progress. His mother was a single parent. Dale did not know his father.

While in the residential treatment center, Dale received intensive treatment that included daily group therapy and weekly individual counseling. He was taught stress management, anger management, and problem-solving and decision-making skills. He also attended a twelve-step group on the center's campus. Dale was put into a behavioral system whereby he could earn increased privileges and freedoms on the residential treatment center campus. He went to school on campus with teachers trained to understand mental health problems. Because the classes were smaller than those found in the typical classroom, he received more individual attention. He was also diagnosed with a reading disorder for which he received help. Dale's problem behaviors improved significantly after six months in the center. Within nine months, he had moved to the least restrictive unit on the campus, allowing him more freedom. For the next three months, he maintained good behavior and utilized the new skills he had learned. After a year in treatment, he was discharged to return home and went back to his old school.

Write your answers to the following questions:

1. What symptoms was Dale experiencing?

2. Does he meet the criteria for either CD or ODD? Explain. If he does, which one?

3. Based on your current knowledge, what interventions would you suggest? Do you believe that the appropriate intervention or treatment was provided?

4. Who should be included in the treatment planning and interventions?

5. What barriers might get in the way of effectively intervening?

6. What suggestions/thoughts/ideas do you have for the other members of Dale's family?

REFERENCES

American Psychiatric Association. (1994). *Diagnostic and statistical manual of mental disorders* (4th ed.). Washington, DC: Author.

American Psychiatric Association. (2013). *Diagnostic and statistical manual of mental disorders* (5th ed.). Washington, DC, Author.

Christensen, A., Phillips, S., Glasgow, R. E., & Johnson, S. M. (1983). Parental characteristics and interactional dysfunction in families with child behavior problems: A preliminary investigation. *Journal of Abnormal Child Psychology, 11,* 153–166.

Dickstein, D. P. (2010). Oppositional defiant disorder. *Journal of the American Academy of Child and Adolescent Psychiatry, 49,* 435–436.

Dumas, J. E., Gibson, J. A., & Albin, J. B. (1989). Behavioral correlates of maternal depressive symptomology in conduct-disordered children. *Journal of Consulting and Clinical Psychology, 57,* 516–521.

Fairchild, G., Passamonti, L., Hurford, G., Hagan, C. C., von dem Hagen, E. A., van Goozen, S. H., . . . Calder, A. J. (2011). Brain structure abnormalities in early-onset and adolescent-onset conduct disorder. *American Journal of Psychiatry, 168,* 624–633.

Fairchild, G., van Goozen, S. H., Calder, A. J., Stollery, S. J., & Goodyer, I. M. (2009). Deficits in facial expression recognition in male adolescents with early-onset or adolescence-onset conduct disorder. *Journal of Child Psychology and Psychiatry, 50,* 627–636.

Fairchild, G., van Goozen, S. H., Stollery, S. J., Aitken, M. R., Savage, J., Moore, S. C., & Goodyer, I. M. (2009). Decision making and executive function in male adolescents with early-onset or adolescence-onset conduct disorder and control subjects. *Biological Psychiatry, 66,* 162–168.

Farmer, E. M. Z., Compton, S. N., Burns, B. J., & Robertson, E. (2002). Review of the evidence base for treatment of childhood psychopathology: Externalizing disorders. *Journal of Consulting and Clinical Psychology, 70,* 1267–1302.

Fergusson, D. M., Lynskey, M. T., & Horwood, L. J. (1993). The effect of maternal depression on maternal ratings of child behavior. *Journal of Abnormal Child Psychology, 21,* 245–269.

Frick, P. J., Lahey, B. B., Loeber, R., Stouthamer-Loeber, M., Christ, M. A. G., & Hanson, K. (1992). Familial risk factors to oppositional defiant disorder and conduct disorder: Parental psychopathological and maternal parenting. *Journal of Consulting and Clinical Psychology, 60,* 49–55.

Henggeler, S. W., Schoenwald, S. K., Borduin, C. M., Rowland, M. D., & Cunningham, P. B. (1998). *Multisystemic treatment of antisocial behavior in children and adolescents.* New York: Guilford Press.

Henggeler, S. W., Schoenwald, S. K., Rowland, M. D., & Cunningham, P. B. (2002). *Serious emotional disturbance in children and adolescents: Multisystemic therapy.* New York: Guilford Press.

Hill, L. G., Coie, J. D., Lochman, J. E., & Greenberg, M. T. (2004). Effectiveness of early screening for externalizing problems: Issues of screening accuracy and utility. *Journal of Consulting and Clinical Psychology, 72,* 809–820.

Marsh, A. A., Finger, E. C., Mitchell, D. G. V., Reid, M. E., Sims, C., Kosson, D. S., . . . Blair, R. J. R. (2008). Reduced amygdala response to fearful expressions in children and adolescents with callous-unemotional traits and disruptive behavior disorders. *American Journal of Psychiatry, 165,* 712–720.

National Institute of Mental Health. (2012). Attention deficit hyperactivity disorder (NIH Publication No. 12–3572). Retrieved from http://www.nimh.nih.gov/health/publica tions/attention-deficit-hyperactivity-disorder/index.shtml

Nigg, J. T., & Hinshaw, S. P. (1998). Parent personality traits and psychopathology associated with antisocial behaviors in childhood attention-deficit hyperactivity disorder. *Journal of Child Psychology and Psychiatry, 39,* 145–159.

Passamonti, L., Fairchild, G., Goodyer, I. M., Hurford, G., Hagan, C. C., Rowe, J. B., & Calder, A. J. (2010). Neural abnormalities in early-onset and adolescence-onset conduct disorder. *Archives of General Psychiatry, 67,* 729–738.

Sterzer, P., Stadler, C., Poustka, F., & Kleinschmidt, A. (2007). A structural neural deficit in adolescents with conduct disorder and its association with lack of empathy. *Neuroimage, 37,* 335–342.

van Goozen, S. H., & Fairchild, G. (2006). Neuroendocrine and neurotransmitter correlates in children with antisocial behavior. *Hormones and Behavior, 50,* 647–654.

van Goozen, S. H., Fairchild, G., Snoek, H., & Harold, G. (2007). The evidence for a
neurobiological model of childhood antisocial behavior. *Psychological Bulletin, 133,*
149–182.

CHAPTER 11

Treatment for Conduct Disorder and Oppositional Defiant Disorder

THE GOOD NEWS IS there are effective interventions in existence for oppositional defiant disorder (ODD) and conduct disorder (CD). However, interventions found to be effective are not effective for everyone. A percentage of the population will not be responsive to these treatments. The earlier the mental health problem is treated, the better the likelihood that the treatment will be successful. That does not mean that intervention with older teenagers who may have been exhibiting the signs and symptoms of one of these disorders for several years will not be effective. Treatment may be more challenging with an older youth, but success is still possible.

Many evidence-based interventions have been highly researched and recognized as evidence-based treatments (EBTs) for both of these externalizing disorders (Burns, Hoagwood, & Mrazek, 1999; Child and Adolescent

Mental Health Division, 2004; Farmer, Compton, Burns, & Robertson, 2002). These EBTs share many of the same components. Many of them use combinations of one or more heavily researched practices found to be effective. These practices may be focused on working individually with caregivers, working with the youth, working with caregivers and youth together, or working with the peer group or community.

EVIDENCE-BASED PRACTICES WITH YOUTH

Practices found to be effective in improving the functioning of youth experiencing CD or ODD are geared toward the youth characteristics often associated with these disorders (Burns et al., 1999; Child and Adolescent Mental Health Division, 2004; Farmer et al., 2002; Waldron & Turner, 2008). Skills training aimed at helping youth identify their normal ways of reacting and learning more effective ways of solving problems or coping with frustrations and the ups and downs of life can help them better maneuver through problems and better adapt to different situations. Because many youth have difficulty with relationships, communication skills and social skills training have been found to be effective in helping them interact more appropriately and positively with peers and authority figures. Self-regulation is another skill that youth can learn to manage their behavior and reduce extreme reactions to minor situations.

Although medication is not a first-line treatment for ODD and CD, it is sometimes prescribed to control some of the more distressing symptoms. Some mental health professionals consider this a form of chemical restraint, meaning that the medication is used to slow the youth down so that they cannot get into as much trouble. Others would consider medication appropriate to treat problems such as aggressive behavior. Either way, medication alone will not be effective in treating ODD or CD. Medication can be effective in treating symptoms related to coexisting conditions such as attention deficit hyperactivity disorder, anxiety, and mood disorders.

EVIDENCE-BASED PRACTICES WITH CAREGIVER(S)

Improving parental management skills in dealing with noncompliant or defiant behavior is a practice that is used across all EBTs for externalizing disorders (Burns et al., 1999; Child and Adolescent Mental Health Division, 2004; Farmer et al., 2002). Well-meaning social workers sometimes tell parents to set boundaries and give consequences for problem behavior. These are things that parents can and should do, but if they are not done correctly or in conjunction with other interventions, the youth's behavior and family functioning can and most likely will get worse. Before a parent disciplines a child, the parent and child must first have positive interactions. Sometimes the first step to changing a youth's problem behavior is to teach a parent to praise and use positive reinforcement for good behavior and to spend time doing something fun with the child. Many people may see this as counterintuitive; however, children are more likely to respond to discipline from someone with whom they have a positive relationship and someone who gives them positive reinforcement for good behaviors.

Providing support for caregivers raising a child with either ODD or CD has been found to be helpful. It can be very difficult for parents/caregivers to deal with extreme problem behaviors. They will need support and understanding. They will also need to learn to take time for themselves doing enjoyable activities and building their own stress-relieving skills. Involving other adults such as a coach can be helpful.

EVIDENCE-BASED PRACTICES WITH YOUTH AND CAREGIVERS TOGETHER

The most effective interventions found for ODD and CD involve a systemic approach. That is, the intervention should not treat only the child or youth; instead, interventions should be focused on all the risk factors discussed in the previous chapter: individual youth characteristics, environmental characteristics, peer group characteristics, and caregiver characteristics (Burns & Hoagwood, 2002; Child and Adolescent Mental Health Division, 2004). If treatment is focused only on the youth and not on other aspects of the youth's life, the intervention will not be either effective or sustaining.

EVIDENCE-BASED TREATMENTS

There are many existing evidence-based treatments geared at externalizing mental health problems. The following are a few of the most heavily researched and disseminated.

Parent-Child Interaction Therapy

Parent-child interaction therapy (PCIT) is a highly researched, evidence-based family intervention for young children age two to seven with behavior disorders. It was developed by Sheila Eyberg based on the idea that optimal parenting and interactions between a caregiver and a child are correlated with better child outcomes (Eyberg, Boggs, & Algina, 1995; Funderburk & Eyberg, 2011). Parent-child interaction therapy uses concepts from play therapy, attachment theory, and social learning theory aimed at teaching caregivers to parent using positive nurturing and appropriate limit setting (authoritative parenting style).

Parent-child interaction therapy consists of two phases. During both phases, the caregiver plays with the child for approximately an hour while the therapist observes the interactions, usually from behind a two-way mirror, and coaches the caregiver, usually through an earpiece. This allows the therapist to witness the caregiver's interactions with the child firsthand and to provide immediate feedback and instruction on better ways to respond. During phase 1 of PCIT (child-directed interaction), the therapist focuses on instructing the caregiver how to interact and respond with the child, with the child as the center of attention. The second phase (parent-directed interaction) focuses on teaching the caregiver effective discipline skills. Through this coaching, caregivers learn strategies for reinforcing their child's positive behaviors and for setting limits without being harsh or negative.

Functional Family Therapy

Functional family therapy (FFT) was developed in 1972 as a strengths-based, family-focused intervention aimed at at-risk youth from ages ten to eighteen who are experiencing acting out behaviors and substance abuse problems, including those diagnosed with ODD or CD (Alexander, Barrett Waldron, Robbins, & Neeb, 2013; Gordon, Graves, & Arbuthnot, 1995). Evaluation of FFT has found it to be highly effective in reducing youth problem behaviors and family conflict, improving family communication, and improving parenting skills. Functional family therapy has been successfully implemented in child welfare, juvenile justice, and mental health service systems. Facilities wanting to be FFT providers must participate in extensive training. Implementation of FFT is highly monitored.

Functional family therapy consists of five major pretreatment and intervention components aimed at reducing risk factors and building protective factors: engagement in change, motivation to change, relational/interpersonal assessment and planning for behavior change, behavior change, and generalization. Therapists work with families for an average of twelve sessions over a three- to four-month period. During the behavior change phase, therapists work with youth and their families on improving communication skills, improving coping, modeling and prompting positive behavior, caregiver parenting skills, and any other area identified as a need.

Multisystemic Therapy

Multisystemic therapy (MST) is an evidence-based intervention that was developed for the treatment of juvenile offenders (Henggeler, 1999, 2003; Henggeler, Melton, Smith, Schoenwald, & Hanley, 1993; Henggeler, Schoenwald, Borduin, Rowland, & Cunningham, 1998; Henggeler, Schoenwald, Rowland, & Cunningham, 2002). It is a community-based treatment that has achieved favorable long-term outcomes to include reduced out-of-home placement and increased school attendance for children and adolescents presenting with serious clinical problems and their families. It takes a social ecological approach to assessment and treatment and utilizes empirically supported goal-oriented treatments, such as cognitive-behavioral therapy, family therapies, or parent training. Assessment focuses on identifying all of the risk factors contributing to a youth's emotional and behavioral problems, and interventions are aimed at all identified sources. Interventions may focus on the youth, caregivers, school environment, peer group, or many other possible influences on the youth's problems.

Multisystemic therapy interventions occur in the youth's natural environment, such as in the home or community, and require active efforts from the caregivers to reach treatment goals. It is the responsibility of the therapist and provider agency to ensure that treatment goals are being met and that families are actively engaged in the treatment process. If goals are not being met, the therapist must reassess the situation, change the treatment strategy, or seek new ways to engage the family.

In order to become an MST provider, an agency must become licensed and agree to adhere to the fidelity of MST. Each MST clinician maintains a caseload of four to six families, allowing time to continuously assess outcomes and provide an intensive level of treatment to the family in its home and community.

Services are problem focused and time limited, lasting from four to six months. The MST therapist or a member of the therapist's team is available twenty-four hours a day, seven days a week, to help the family work through any crisis that may arise. An on-site supervisor provides regularly scheduled weekly clinical supervision to the MST team and monitors the therapist's adherence to MST fidelity. In addition to on-site supervision, each MST team and supervisor works closely with an assigned consultant from MST Services who monitors MST fidelity and helps the team overcome treatment barriers and develop treatment strategies. More information on MST or how to become a certified provider can be found at http://mstservices.com.

Multidimensional Treatment Foster Care

Multidimensional treatment foster care (MTFC) is an evidence-based treatment that was developed as a cost-effective alternative to regular foster care placements, residential treatment, or incarceration of youth who have severe behavior problems (Leve, Fisher, & Chamberlain, 2009; Westermark, Hansson, & Olsson, 2011). Early evidence suggests that it is effective in reducing substance abuse among teenagers as well (Smith, Chamberlain, & Eddy, 2010). Youth are placed in foster homes with highly trained and well-supported foster parents for approximately six to nine months. While youth are in the placement, they receive skills training, supportive therapy, school-based behavioral interventions, and supportive mentoring. The foster parents implement a structured plan that has been designed by a program supervisor with input from a treatment team consisting of a family therapist, an individual therapist, and a child skills trainer.

The biological family (or other caregiver) receives supportive family therapy to prepare for the youth's return to the home and parenting skills training to learn to provide close supervision, set fair and consistent limits, and provide consistent consequences for problem behaviors. The caregiver and youth have sessions and home visits together to allow the caregiver time to practice skills and receive feedback before the youth returns home permanently. Multidimensional treatment foster care can only be provided by programs that are certified or are receiving clinical supervision from TFC Consultants, Inc.

CASE STUDIES

Let's return to the case studies of the youth from chapter 10. You will see the diagnosis and any additional interventions that they received. Finally, you will see the outcome for each youth.

Tim

Tim is the thirteen-year-old boy living with his mother and eleven-year-old sister in a public housing apartment complex. His father is deceased and his mother has an intellectual disability with an IQ under 90. Tim and his sister both have normal IQs.

Tim refused to listen to his mother and tormented his sister. He had several encounters with the juvenile justice system. He was adjudicated as a sex offender and started counseling. He re-offended and was ordered into an inpatient sex offender treatment program where he received intensive individual and group therapy. Tim was diagnosed with conduct disorder. When he was released from the sex offender treatment program, he returned home with his mother and sister. He remained on probation under a specialized probation unit. He is now fifteen years old and his sister is thirteen.

When Tim first returned home, there was a honeymoon period. He followed his mother's rules and left his sister alone. As time passed, Tim began to pick up the delinquent behavior he exhibited prior to his adjudication. He ignored his mother's requests. His probation officer met with him weekly. If Tim missed the curfew set by the judge or skipped school, his probation officer sent him to juvenile detention. Tim re-offended by sexually abusing a seven-year-old neighbor. He was sentenced by a judge to remain in a state juvenile facility until he turned eighteen.

Tracy

Tracy is the eight-year-old girl who was exhibiting negative and acting out behavior. She got in trouble at school, talking back to her teachers and sometimes refusing to do her work. The other children in her classes did not like her because she was a bully. She did not always follow the rules at home. Tracy often screamed and yelled, ran to her room, and slammed the door. Tracy's parents were at their wits' end. Her mother took her to see a counselor. The counselor diagnosed Tracy with oppositional defiant disorder. Tracy attended therapy for an hour each week, working with her therapist on anger management, coping, and problem-solving and social skills. After a few months, there were no noticeable changes in Tracy's behaviors at school or home. The therapist discharged Tracy from treatment.

Over the next two years, Tracy continued to exhibit behavioral problems. Once again at her wits' end, Tracy's mother sought help. The family was referred to receive wraparound treatment. Tracy and her parents, with guidance from the facilitator, helped to decide who they wanted to include on their family team. Team members initially included Tracy, her parents, a younger sister, a school-teacher, and her mother's best friend, whom Tracy really liked. The wraparound facilitator guided the team through a process of identifying the family's strengths and needs and developing a wraparound plan (service plan). The team identified formal and informal community services and supports to address the needs of the child and family. Tracy's parents received help with their parenting skills twice a week in their own home from a trained therapist. Her mother started attending a support group with other parents of children experiencing problems similar to Tracy's.

Tracy's teacher helped implement a behavior plan at school whereby Tracy could earn time to play video games or do other things she enjoyed. A daily report was e-mailed to Tracy's parents. If she had a good report, she was allowed to stay up and watch television for an extra thirty minutes. If she had a bad day, she was not allowed to watch her favorite shows that night.

Tracy started equestrian therapy in which she was assigned a horse to groom, feed, and ride a couple of times a week. As part of the therapy, she learned how to take responsibility for her actions and problem solving and coping skills. Tracy loved riding and taking care of the horse. Her self-esteem improved. She also attended a weekly skills training group with other children. Tracy's behaviors changed considerably. She made a friend at school with whom she ate lunch and had sleepovers.

James

James is the seventeen-year-old who lived with his parents in a middle class neighborhood. He was afraid of his father's explosive anger, but intimidated his mother when his father was at work. James hung out with a group of peers who abused drugs and alcohol. He was a bully to others. James was placed in detention for three months after he severely beat his mother, landing her in the hospital. He was diagnosed with conduct disorder while in detention. He was discharged to return home with strict orders from the judge that he would be sent to a more restrictive lockup facility until he turned twenty-one if he did not comply with his probation or had any more incidents of trouble. His family was offered MST; the parents agreed, but James was not so agreeable.

The MST therapist worked mostly with James's parents, helping them to manage James's behaviors. James refused to speak with the therapist. The therapist worked with his parents on being partners in dealing with James's behaviors and worked with his father on managing his own explosive temper. The family learned how to spend positive time together and they incorporated a family dinner night on Sunday evenings.

James was very negative and continued to be defiant for the first two months of MST. As part of his probation, he was ordered not to hang out with his old friends, to attend school regularly, and not to use drugs or alcohol. His probation officer worked with the MST therapist and his parents to enforce the rules. He tested James for drug use on an intermittent basis. He put James on an ankle monitor for breaking curfew and hanging out with his old friends.

The MST therapist worked with James and his parents to develop a behavior plan. James loved listening to hard rock and had always wanted to play guitar. A behavioral plan was set up whereby James could earn a new electric guitar and lessons that would be purchased through flexible funds offered as a component of MST. James was able to earn the guitar and lessons. Through the music studio where he took lessons, he met some other guys and they started a band. James's behavior at home and school completely changed. The MST therapist stopped working with the family after five months. The next summer, James's mother sent a thank you letter to the MST therapist. James graduated from high school. His behaviors had changed and he was enrolled in a technical school.

Dale

Dale is the sixteen-year-old who was placed in residential care for a year. He was diagnosed with conduct disorder. While he was in care, his parents had limited participation in treatment other than a monthly meeting with the social worker to discuss his progress. Dale received intensive treatment and skills training. Dale was put on a behavioral system whereby he could earn increased privileges and freedoms on the residential treatment center campus. He went to school on campus with teachers trained to understand mental health problems. Within nine months, Dale's behaviors improved to the point where he was moved to the least restrictive unit on the campus, allowing him more freedom. After a year in treatment, he was discharged to return home and went back to his old school.

When Dale returned home, he utilized his new skills and did his best to follow rules and do well in school. His mother was very harsh and her reactions were unpredictable. Dale felt that, no matter what he did, his mother would yell or hit him. In the larger classroom setting, he began to struggle to keep up with others. Within six months, he was back to getting in trouble, using drugs, and hanging out with his old friends. He stole a car and ended up back in the detention center. As an alternative to sending him back to the residential treatment center or keeping him locked up in the detention center, he and his mother were referred to a multimodal treatment foster care pilot being implemented using grant funding. He was placed in a foster home with trained foster parents in his community. This time, both he and his mother received help together and individually. An advocate helped get him into the correct educational setting. His mother was referred to a psychiatrist who diagnosed her with bipolar disorder and prescribed a mood stabilizer. She received skills training to help her better cope with stress and anxiety. After three months, Dale began having home visits. After six months, he returned home to live with his mother and was reportedly doing well.

Consider the following questions:

1. What do these real life scenarios have in common?

2. What are the differences?

3. Now that you have learned what happened to each of the youths, do you have any different thoughts on how you would have handled the situation if you were the families' social worker?

REFERENCES

Alexander, J. F., Barrett Waldron, H., Robbins, M. S., & Neeb, A. A. (2013). *Functional family therapy for adolescent behavior problems.* Washington, DC: American Psychological Association.

Burns, B. J., & Hoagwood, K. (Eds.). (2002). *Community treatment for youth: Evidence-based interventions for severe emotional and behavioral disorders.* New York: Oxford University Press.

Burns, B. J., Hoagwood, K., & Mrazek, P. J. (1999). Effective treatment for mental disorders in children and adolescents. *Clinical Child and Family Psychology Review, 2,* 199–254.

Child and Adolescent Mental Health Division. (2004). *Evidence-based Service Committee—Biennial report—Summary of effective interventions for youth with behavioral and emotional needs.* Honolulu: Hawaii Department of Health.

Eyberg, S., Boggs, S., & Algina, J. (1995). Parent-child interaction therapy: A psycho-social model for the treatment of young children with conduct problem behavior and their families. *Psychopharmacology Bulletin, 3*, 83–91.

Farmer, E. M. Z., Compton, S. N., Burns, B. J., & Robertson, E. (2002). Review of the evidence base for treatment of childhood psychopathology: Externalizing disorders. *Journal of Consulting and Clinical Psychology, 70*, 1267–1302.

Funderburk, B. W., & Eyberg, S. (2011). Parent–child interaction therapy. In J. C. Norcross, G. R. VandenBos, & D. K. Freedheim (Eds.), *History of psychotherapy: Continuity and change* (2nd ed., pp. 415–420). Washington, DC: American Psychological Association.

Gordon, D., Graves, K., & Arbuthnot, J. (1995). The effect of functional family therapy for delinquents on adult criminal behavior. *Criminal Justice and Behavior, 22*, 60–73. doi:10.1177/0093854895022001005

Henggeler, S. W. (1999). Multisystemic therapy: An overview of clinical procedures, outcomes, and policy implications. *Child Psychology and Psychiatry Review, 4*, 4–9.

Henggeler, S. W. (2003). Multisystemic therapy: An evidence-based practice for serious clinical problems in adolescents. *NAMI Beginnings, 3*, Fall, 8–10.

Henggeler, S. W., Melton, G. B., Smith, L. A., Schoenwald, S. K., & Hanley, J. H. (1993). Family preservation using multisystemic treatment: Long-term follow-up to a clinical trial with serious juvenile offenders. *Journal of Child and Family Studies, 2*, 283–293.

Henggeler, S. W., Schoenwald, S. K., Borduin, C. M., Rowland, M. D., & Cunningham, P. B. (1998). *Multisystemic treatment of antisocial behavior in children and adolescents*. New York: Guilford Press.

Henggeler, S. W., Schoenwald, S. K., Rowland, M. D., & Cunningham, P. B. (2002). *Serious emotional disturbance in children and adolescents: Multisystemic therapy*. New York: Guilford Press.

Leve, L., Fisher, P., & Chamberlain, P. (2009). Multidimensional treatment foster care as a preventive intervention to promote resiliency among youth in the child welfare system. *Journal of Personality, 77*, 6.

Smith, D., Chamberlain, P., & Eddy, M. (2010). Preliminary support for multidimensional treatment foster care in reducing substance use in delinquent boys. *Journal of Child & Adolescent Substance Abuse, 19*, 343–358.

Waldron, H. B., & Turner, C. W. (2008). Evidence-based psychosocial treatments for adolescent substance abuser. *Journal of Clinical Child and Adolescent Psychology, 37*, 238–261.

Westermark, P. K., Hansson, K., & Olsson, M. (2011). Multidimensional treatment foster care (MTFC): Results from an independent replication. *Journal of Family Therapy, 33*, 20–41. doi:10.1111/j.1467–6427.2010.00515.x

CHAPTER 12

Bipolar Disorder

Bipolar disorder, also known as manic depression, is a category of mood disorders known as bipolar I, bipolar II, bipolar not otherwise specified (NOS), and cyclothymia (American Psychiatric Association, 2000, 2013). Bipolar disorder is a brain disorder that results in unusual changes in a person's mood and energy level. As its name implies, it is characterized by extreme highs (mania) and/or extreme lows (major depression, as discussed in chapter 4). Between episodes, some people experience lingering symptoms whereas others may be symptom free (Goodwin & Jamison, 2007). Bipolar disorder is prevalent in approximately 2.6 percent of the population. It is thought to affect about 7 percent of children who receive psychiatric treatment (Brotman et al., 2006). There is currently no cure for bipolar disorder. We hope that the ongoing research on bipolar disorder will someday result in a cure. For now, it is a lifelong illness. However, with treatment people can recover and live happy, healthy, productive lives (Kessler et al., 2005; National Depressive and Manic-Depressive Association, 2001).

SIGNS AND SYMPTOMS

Mania and Hypomania

Mania is far more extreme than the emotion that a person would normally expect to experience when happy or excited. Mania causes serious problems to the point that it interferes with a person's ability to function in daily life. According to the *DSM*, symptoms of mania include:

- Excessive energy, restlessness, racing thoughts, and rapid talking;
- Denial that anything is wrong;
- Extremely happy feelings;
- Being easily irritated;
- Little need for sleep;
- Unrealistic belief in one's ability;
- Poor judgment;
- Sustained, unusual behavior;
- Increased sex drive;
- Substance abuse;
- Aggressive behavior;
- Paranoia.

During a manic episode, someone may go days without needing any sleep or may be overly restless. The person may experience excessive energy and do things such as clean the entire house from top to bottom for hours on end. Poor judgment, increased sex drive, and extreme risk-taking behaviors have also been found to accompany mania. Any of these issues alone can be a serious problem. Someone in a manic episode may be overly sexually promiscuous, putting him or her at high risk of contracting a sexually transmitted disease or experiencing an unwanted pregnancy. It is not uncommon for adults to go on wild spending sprees and max out their credit cards or credit cards stolen from others, purchasing things they do not need and leaving themselves or someone else in significant debt.

Delusional thinking and inflated self-esteem are often symptoms of mania. Some persons experiencing a manic episode truly believe that they are famous movie stars, members of royalty, or excellent singers. Some adults have been known to suddenly fly to another country, believing that they are being sent there for some special purpose. At other times, they may be extremely irritable for no reason or show unusual behavior for an extended period of time. Aggressive behavior, substance abuse, and extreme feelings of paranoia are other common symptoms. At the end of a manic episode, a person experiences a *crash*. Some people describe their crash as the end of good times. Many report feeling on top of the world, as if they can do anything, immediately followed by waking up and being unable to function. They have expended all their energy. Mania can feel exhilarating and exciting; going into the crash can feel as if one has fallen into a black hole of sadness and despair that will never end.

Hypomania is similar to mania, but symptoms that accompany it are not as intense and not as disruptive to daily life. There is a clear difference from a person's normal mood that persists for at least four days. The change in mood may present as persistently elevated or persistently irritable. Psychotic symptoms do not occur with hypomania.

When experiencing an exhilarated mood, a person can feel quite good and not perceive the hypomania as a problem. People often describe the feeling as being high. They experience excessive energy. Ideas come faster. They may feel more creative, more confident, less shy, and/or more productive. If not treated, a hypomanic episode may transform into a severe manic or depressive episode (Goodwin & Jamison, 2007).

CAUSES

The causes of bipolar disorder are not completely known; however, there does seem to be evidence that the cause includes a combined genetic, environmental, and biochemical relationship. Bipolar disorder has been found to run in families (Lin et al., 2006). Children who have a parent or other close relative with bipolar disorder are more likely to develop it than children with no family history of the disorder (Nurnberger & Foroud, 2000). Some estimates report that as many as 4 to 24 percent of persons who have a first degree biological relative with bipolar I, 1 to 5 percent of persons with a first degree relative with bipolar II, and 4 to 24 percent of persons with a first degree relative with major depression also have bipolar disorder. Studies of twins and adoptions provide strong evidence of a genetic connection to bipolar disorder, but they also suggest that environment plays a role.

Research has found that bipolar I and bipolar II are equally likely to occur among different races, ethnicities, and genders (Gonzalez et al., 2007; Manchia et al., 2008). In bipolar I, males are more likely to experience mania as a first symptom. Females are more likely to experience major depression as a first symptom. Women are at risk of developing symptoms following birth, particularly psychotic symptoms. Sometimes women will experience their first episode of mania or major depression postpartum. This episode often includes psychosis. When a woman is premenstrual, she can experience a worsening of manic or depressive symptoms. Emerging research suggests that bipolar II is more common in women than in men. Women experience more major depressive symptoms than men through the course of the disease. Men are more prone to hypomania than depression. They experience as many or more hypomanic episodes as major depressive episodes.

Several studies show that youth with anxiety or major depressive disorders are more likely to develop bipolar disorder than youth who never experience these disorders (Krishnan, 2005; Mueser et al., 1998). Youth who experience multiple recurrences of major depression are 10 to 15 percent more likely to develop bipolar I disorder than are other youth (Bellivier et al., 2003; Bellivier, Golmard, Henry, Leboyer, & Schurhoff, 2001). Although those who experience an anxiety or depressive disorder are at higher risk of developing bipolar disorder than persons in the general population, it must be noted that the majority of children and teens with anxiety disorders do not develop bipolar disorder.

Drug and alcohol abuse has been found to occur in more than half of people diagnosed with bipolar disorder (Bizzarri et al., 2007; Strakowski et al., 1998). If a youth is predisposed to bipolar disorder, abusing drugs or alcohol can increase the likelihood of developing it. Sometimes youth experience symptoms of bipolar disorder and use alcohol or drugs in order to feel normal. This is called self-medicating.

BIPOLAR DISORDER AND THE BRAIN

Bipolar spectrum disorders are considered brain disorders. Scientists have been studying the brain in an effort to find the biological correlates to bipolar disorder.

As discussed previously, norepinephrine, serotonin, and dopamine are the neuro-transmitters that are involved in the functioning of the brain and body. Research suggests that abnormalities in serotonin and dopamine are contributors to bipolar disorder (Soares & Mann, 1997a, 1997b). Ongoing studies have found that the brain of a child with bipolar disorder does not perform in the same ways as it does in healthy children (Gogtay et al., 2007; Soares & Mann, 1997a, 1997b). Through a noninvasive technique that allows scientists to measure brain functioning (magnetoencephalography), differences between children with bipolar disorder and other children have been found in the areas of the brain that direct attention to identify environmental signals and that organize behavior. Imaging studies have helped identify different brain activity patterns and connections associated with the symptoms of bipolar disorder. For instance, children with bipolar disorder have been found to have difficulty in identifying facial expressions in others. It is believed by the scientific community that this may be an inherited trait that affects children with bipolar disorder and other children who have a first degree relative with the disorder. A link between bipolar disorder and altered genes has also been found. The altered gene that seems to have the most correlation with bipolar disorder is located in the axons in a region of the brain responsible for controlling the firing of neurons. As science continues to advance our knowledge of bipolar disorder, it will allow for preventative interventions, improved treatments, and someday a cure.

DIAGNOSING BIPOLAR DISORDER

The diagnosis of bipolar disorder is based on patient self-reports and reports from family members or other persons who have witnessed abnormal behavior. In addition to the psychiatric evaluation, a physical exam, including a complete laboratory panel, should be conducted to rule out a general medical condition or substance abuse as the underlying cause of symptoms.

As stated above, bipolar disorder is really a category of mood disorders rather than one singular disorder. The commonality across these categories is the presence of one or more incidents of an abnormally elevated energy level, called mania or hypomania. Depending on the type of bipolar disorder a person develops, he or she may experience depressive episodes as well. Both manic and depressive episodes are often separated by periods of normal mood that can last weeks, months, or even years in some persons. For some persons, depression and mania may rapidly alternate, a condition known as *rapid cycling*. In addition to the types and intensities of symptoms experienced, a key factor in meeting the criteria for bipolar disorder is that the symptoms cause significant distress or impairment across daily functioning. With the exception of a few changes in wording, the categories and diagnostic criteria for bipolar disorder have not changed from *DSM-IV* (American Psychiatric Association, 1994) to *DSM-5* (American Psychiatric Association, 2013).

Bipolar I

To meet the criteria for bipolar I, a person must have experienced one or more manic episodes. With bipolar I, experiencing a depressive episode is not required for the diagnosis; however, depressive episodes frequently occur.

Bipolar II

Bipolar II disorder is characterized by a history or occurrence of a hypomanic episode and at least one episode meeting the criteria for major depression. Hypomania is characterized by the same symptoms as mania, such as increased energy, but in less extreme forms. Because of this, bipolar II is more difficult to diagnose than bipolar I. Hypomania can appear similar to a period of successful, high productivity; thus, it is less likely to be reported than depressive episodes.

Cyclothymia

Cyclothymia is characterized by a presence or history of hypomanic episodes with periods of depression that do not meet criteria for major depressive episodes. A diagnosis of cyclothymia requires the presence of numerous hypomanic episodes intermingled with depressive episodes. A person with cyclothymia experiences more moderate cycling of moods. These mood changes interfere with a person's functioning, but they appear to the observer to be a personality trait.

BIPOLAR DISORDER IN CHILDREN AND TEENS

Not that long ago, bipolar disorder was believed to emerge in late adolescence or adulthood. Although symptoms of bipolar disorder more often emerge after childhood, it is now recognized that they can begin in early childhood. Children as young as six years old are being diagnosed with bipolar disorder, and prevalence rates of bipolar in adolescents are close to those found in adults.

There is debate among health care providers and others as to whether the increased prevalence of bipolar disorder in children and young teens is accurate or whether it is being wrongly or overly diagnosed. On one side of the argument, it is believed that children are finally being accurately diagnosed because mental health professionals are more knowledgeable of the disorder in children. Those making this argument assert that earlier identification leads to earlier appropriate treatment that can result in a better trajectory of the disorder.

The other side of the argument is that bipolar disorder is being overdiagnosed in children and teenagers. People in this camp believe it to be the latest fad in psychiatry rather than accurate early diagnosis. Some in this camp believe that we as a society are using bipolar disorder as a crutch or a label to explain away inappropriate behaviors that would have been dealt with through discipline in the past. The answer to this debate probably lies somewhere in the middle. What is known is that children can develop bipolar disorder, and if it is identified and treated early, they can experience better outcomes and functioning.

Research suggests that persons who begin experiencing symptoms of bipolar disorder during early childhood have more severe symptoms and a poorer trajectory of the disorder than those who begin experiencing symptoms in early adulthood (Bellivier et al., 2001; Carter, Mundo, Parikh, & Kennedy, 2003; Hamshere et al., 2009; Kessler et al., 2005; Perlis et al., 2004). Hamshere and colleagues report that in early childhood children are more likely to experience manic symptoms and rapid mood cycling. These cycles are seen as unpredictable, alternating between behavior that is aggressive and behavior that is silly. A child may appear to have an extremely short temper at times or experience unusually irritable moods, resulting in explosive temper tantrums or rages that may last several hours. These are not the normal silliness or irritability that a child would ordinarily experience. Younger children who develop bipolar disorder often experience audio and visual hallucinations. Other common symptoms of early onset bipolar disorder in young children include:

- Bed wetting (especially in boys)
- Night terrors
- Rapid or pressured speech
- Obsessional behavior

- Excessive daydreaming
- Compulsive behavior
- Motor and vocal tics
- Learning disabilities
- Poor short-term memory
- Lack of organization
- Fascination with gore or morbid topics
- Hypersexuality
- Manipulative behavior
- Bossiness
- Lying
- Suicidal thoughts
- Destruction of property
- Paranoia

Although children and adolescents can experience the same symptoms as adults, they often experience symptoms that present differently than in adults. This makes diagnosing bipolar disorder in children and adolescents more difficult than diagnosing it in adults. Many of the symptoms are common to other mental health disorders experienced by youth such as attention deficit hyperactivity disorder (ADHD) or oppositional defiant disorder (ODD). The symptoms can also be mistaken for normal adolescent moodiness. If a child is misdiagnosed as having ADHD or depression, depending on the symptoms, there can be dangerous consequences. Someone predisposed to bipolar disorder who takes the stimulant Ritalin or an antidepressant such as Prozac or Zoloft can experience extreme manic and/or psychotic behaviors. Accurate diagnosis is imperative. It should also be noted that children may start out with symptoms of one type of bipolar disorder and later switch to symptoms of another type of the disorder (Birmaher et al., 2006).

Youth experiencing mania may become easily distracted, hyper, and/or impulsive, which can appear more like ADHD. Severe acting out and aggressive behaviors can appear to be an oppositional disorder. Behaviors may seem erratic and oppositional. Youth often take risks without thinking because their thoughts are moving really fast, not allowing them time to consider the consequences. They may also feel indestructible and supreme. Common risk-taking behavior includes drug and alcohol use, dangerous stunts, and illegal behavior. An increased sex drive or obsession with sex can be a symptom of mania. Coupling that with risk-taking behavior can result in the youth having unprotected sex.

Both manic and depressive symptoms can interfere with school performance. For youth experiencing mania, the risk taking, impulsiveness, and erratic behaviors can become disciplinary problems. Racing thoughts and inability to concentrate interfere with the ability to focus on work. Relationships with peers are very likely to become problematic. The inability to comprehend others' facial expressions can lead to misunderstanding of social cues and can be a recipe for getting into arguments and fights.

Disruptive Mood Dysregulation Disorder

A new diagnostic category called disruptive mood dysregulation disorder (DMDD) has been added to the *DSM-5* to capture youth who experience significant difficulties such as severe temper outbursts and extreme irritability, but do not have the classic symptoms such as mania/hypomania or characteristics such as a family history of bipolar disorder. The symptoms of both bipolar disorder and ODD have many similarities with DMDD; however, there are distinct differences as well (American Psychiatric Association, 2013). It is the distinct differences between the disorders that prompted research resulting in the addition of the new diagnosis. Youth with ODD exhibit extreme defiant behavior directed toward persons in authority; however, the duration and intensity do not meet the same threshold as the symptoms associated with DMDD. Disruptive mood dysregulation disorder differs from bipolar disorder in that the symptoms are constant rather than episodic. The symptoms of DMDD occur at least two to three times a week and last for at least a year. Many youth who fit into this new diagnostic category are those who were historically being diagnosed with bipolar disorder not otherwise specified (NOS) because they were experiencing extreme problems that did not meet the criteria for ODD or bipolar disorder. The criteria listed in the *DSM-5* (American Psychiatric Association, 2013) for DMDD include the following:

1. Severe recurrent temper outbursts that are grossly out of proportion, in intensity or duration, to the situation.
   a. The temper outbursts are manifested verbally and/or behaviorally, such as in the form of verbal rages or physical aggression toward people or property.

      b.   The temper outbursts are inconsistent with developmental level.

2.   The temper outbursts occur, on average, three or more times per week.

3.   An irritable or angry mood is exhibited between temper outbursts:
      a.   Nearly every day, for most of the day, the mood between temper outbursts is persistently irritable or angry.
      b.   The irritable or angry mood is observable by others (e.g., parents, teachers, and peers).

4.   Criteria 1–3 have been present for twelve or more months without three or more consecutive months without the symptoms of criteria 1–3.

5.   Criterion 1 or 3 is present in at least two settings (at home, at school, or with peers) and must be severe in at least one setting.

6.   The diagnosis should not be made for the first time before age six or after age eighteen.

7.   The onset of criteria 1 through 5 is before the age of ten.

8.   There has never been a distinct period lasting more than one day during which an abnormally elevated or expansive mood was present most of the day, and the abnormally elevated or expansive mood was accompanied by the onset, or worsening, of mania.

9.   The behaviors do not occur exclusively during an episode of major depressive disorder and are not better accounted for by another mental disorder. The symptoms are not due to the effects of a drug or to a general medical or neurological condition.

CASE STUDIES

Following are some case studies of youth with symptoms similar to those discussed in this chapter. Chapter 13 will explore evidence-based treatments and practices for bipolar disorder. We will then return to the case studies presented in this chapter to learn of the actual interventions provided.

Tina

Tina is a thirteen-year-old who always made good grades, had lots of friends, and loved sports. Her behavior suddenly changed. She began having trouble sleeping, often pacing around the house throughout the night. She was unable to sleep more than two hours a night for several days, but she claimed to not feel tired.

At times her mood was overly happy and the next minute it seemed angry and irritable. She would curse at others for no known reason. She started talking rapidly about a lot of different things, but mainly she boasted about how much smarter and more popular she was than everyone else. During school, her behaviors were very disruptive. She would talk over the teacher about things not related to the class.

Her parents became concerned that she was using drugs. They did not know how to handle the situation. The final straw for them was when she stole their car and went for a ride even though she was not old enough to drive. The police stopped her for speeding. When they learned that she was not old enough to drive, they took her to the juvenile detention center. Her parents were able to convince the judge to drop the charges and allow them to take her to a hospital for drug and alcohol treatment.

When Tina was taken in for treatment, the doctor ordered a toxicology screening to determine what drugs she had been taking. Tina denied using drugs or alcohol. Her toxicology report came back negative for drugs and alcohol. She was transferred to the psychiatric adolescent unit of the hospital, and with parental consent, was started on Depakote against her will. Her parents did not want her to take the medication, but they did not know what else to do. After spending three weeks in the hospital, Tina was discharged and returned home to her normal life and school. She was given a follow-up appointment with her psychiatrist.

Consider the following questions:

1. What symptoms was Tina experiencing?
2. Does she meet the criteria for a bipolar diagnosis? Explain. If she does, which one?
3. Based on your current knowledge, what interventions would you suggest? Do you believe that the appropriate intervention or treatment was provided?

4. Who should be included in the treatment planning and interventions?

5. What barriers might get in the way of effectively intervening?

6. What suggestions/thoughts/ideas do you have for the other members of her family?

Jack

When Jack was seven years old, his parents noticed changes in his mood and behaviors over the course of several months. One minute, he would act silly and say silly things. He would make weird faces, laugh hysterically out of the clear blue, and run around the house. The next minute he would begin crying and tell his parents that he hated himself because he was ugly and stupid. He would apologize over and over for things that he perceived he did wrong, but in reality these were of no consequence. He went through periods of not needing sleep and exhibiting an extreme level of energy. During these times, he would start an activity and then move on to another activity without finishing the first. At other times, he would isolate himself in his room and not show any interest in playing video games or playing with friends. He would hit his baby sister, punch a wall, or exhibit other unprovoked aggressive behaviors. He told his parents he did these things because the voices were telling him to do bad things.

Jack's parents became frustrated with Jack's behavior, believing he was doing these things to get attention. Punishment did not seem to change his behaviors. One day, he choked his baby sister, bruising her neck. His mother called the police. The police said that they could not do anything to help because Jack was only seven years old; they told her to call social services because he was a danger to his sister. Social services helped the parents find a residential facility, where Jack was admitted for long-term care.

Write your answers to the following questions:

1. What symptoms was Jack experiencing?

2. Does he meet the criteria for a bipolar diagnosis? Explain. If he does, which one?

3. Based on your current knowledge, what interventions would you suggest? Do you believe that the appropriate intervention or treatment (if any) was provided?

4. Who should be included in the treatment planning and interventions?
5. What barriers might get in the way of effectively intervening?
6. What suggestions/thoughts/ideas do you have for members of his family?

REFERENCES

American Psychiatric Association. (1994). *Diagnostic and statistical manual of mental disorders* (4th ed.). Washington, DC: Author.

American Psychiatric Association. (2000). *Diagnostic and statistical manual of mental disorders* (4th ed., text rev.). Washington, DC: Author.

American Psychiatric Association. (2013). *Diagnostic and statistical manual of mental disorders* (5th ed.). Washington, DC, Author.

Bellivier, F., Golmard, J. L., Henry, C., Leboyer, M., & Schurhoff, F. (2001). Admixture analysis of age at onset in bipolar I affective disorder. *Archives of General Psychiatry, 58,* 510–512.

Bellivier, F., Golmard, J. L., Rietschel, M., Schultze, T. G., Malafosse, A., Preisig, M., . . . Lebover, M. (2003). Age at onset in bipolar I affective disorder: Further evidence for three subgroups. *American Journal of Psychiatry, 160,* 999–1001.

Birmaher, B., Axelson, D., Strober, M., Gill, M. K., Valeri, S., Chiappetta, L., . . . Keller, M. (2006). Clinical course of children and adolescents with bipolar spectrum disorders. *Archives of General Psychiatry, 63,* 175–183.

Bizzarri, J. V., Sbrana, A., Rucci, P., Ravani, L., Massei, G. J., Gonnelli, C., . . . Cassano, G. B. (2007). The spectrum of substance abuse in bipolar disorder: Reasons for use, sensation seeking and substance sensitivity. *Bipolar Disorder, 9,* 213–220.

Brotman, M. A., Schmajuk, M., Rich, B. A., Dickstein, D. P., Guyer, A. E., Costello, E. J., . . . Leibenluft, E. (2006). Prevalence, clinical correlates, and longitudinal course of severe mood dysregulation in children. *Biological Psychiatry, 60,* 991–997.

Carter, T. D., Mundo, E., Parikh, S. V., & Kennedy, J. L. (2003). Early age at onset as a risk factor for poor outcome of bipolar disorder. *Journal of Psychiatric Residency, 37,* 297–303.

Gogtay, N., Ordonez, A., Herman, D. H., Hayashi, K. M., Greenstein, D., Vaituzis, C., . . . Rapoport, J. L. (2007). Dynamic mapping of cortical development before and after the onset of pediatric bipolar illness. *Journal of Child Psychology and Psychiatry, 48,* 852–862.

Gonzalez, J. M., Thompson, P., Escamilla, M., Araga, M., Singh, V., Farrelly, N., . . . Bowden, C. L. (2007). Treatment characteristics and illness burden among European Americans, African Americans, and Latinos in the first 2,000 patients of the systematic treatment enhancement program for bipolar disorder. *Psychopharmacological Bulletin, 40,* 31–46.

Goodwin, F. K., & Jamison, K. R. (2007). *Manic-depressive illness: Bipolar disorders and recurrent depression* (2nd ed.). New York: Oxford University Press.

Hamshere, M. L., Gordon-Smith, K., Forty, L., Jones, L., Caesar, S., Fraser, C., . . . Smith, D. J. (2009). Age-at-onset in bipolar-I disorder: Mixture analysis of 1369 cases identifies three distinct clinical sub-groups. *Journal of Affective Disorders, 116,* 23–29.

Kessler, R. C., Berglund, P., Demler, O., Jin, R., Merikangas, K. R., & Walters, E. E. (2005). Lifetime prevalence and age-of-onset distributions of DSM-IV disorders in the National Comorbidity Survey Replication. *Archives of General Psychiatry, 62,* 593–602.

Krishnan, K. R. (2005). Psychiatric and medical comorbidities of bipolar disorder. *Psychosomatic Medicine, 67*(1), 1–8.

Lin, P. I., McInnis, M. G., Potash, J. B., Willour, V., MacKinnon, D. F., DePaulo, R., & Zandi, P. P. (2006). Clinical correlates and familial aggregation of age at onset in bipolar disorder. *American Journal of Psychiatry, 163,* 240–246.

Manchia, M., Lampus, S., Chillotti, C., Sardu, C., Ardau, R., Severino, G., & Del Zompo, M. (2008). Age at onset in Sardinian bipolar I patients: Evidence for three subgroups. *Bipolar Disorders, 10,* 443–446.

Mueser, K. T., Goodman, L. B., Trumbetta, S. L., Rosenberg, S. D., Osher, C., Vidaver, F. C., . . . Foy, D. W. (1998). Trauma and posttraumatic stress disorder in severe mental illness. *Journal of Consulting and Clinical Psychology, 66,* 493–499.

National Depressive and Manic-Depressive Association. (2001). *Living with bipolar disorder: How far have we really come?* [Community survey]. Retrieved from http://www.dbsalliance.org/pdfs/bphowfar1.pdf

Nurnberger, J. I., Jr., & Foroud, T. (2000). Genetics of bipolar affective disorder. *Current Psychiatry Reports, 2,* 147–157.

Perlis, R. H., Miyahara, S., Marangell, L. B., Wisniewski, S. R., Ostacher, M., DelBello, M. P., . . . Nierenberg, A. A. (2004). Long-term implications of early onset in bipolar disorder: Data from the first 1000 participants in the systematic treatment enhancement program for bipolar disorder (STEP-BD). *Biological Psychiatry, 55,* 875–881.

Soares, J. C., & Mann, J. J. (1997a). The anatomy of mood disorders—Review of structural neuroimaging studies. *Biological Psychiatry, 41,* 86–106.

Soares, J. C., & Mann, J. J. (1997b). The functional neuroanatomy of mood disorders. *Journal of Psychiatric Residency, 31,* 393–432.

Strakowski, S. M., Sax, K. W., McElroy, S. L., Keck, P. E., Jr., Hawkins, J. M., & West, S. A. (1998). Course of psychiatric and substance abuse syndromes co-occurring with bipolar disorder after a first psychiatric hospitalization. *Journal of Consulting and Clinical Psychology, 59,* 465–471.

CHAPTER 13

Treatment of Bipolar Disorder

As with other mental health disorders discussed in this book, there is currently no cure for bipolar disorder. However, people can recover through treatment and lead a normal life. Treatment focuses on controlling and preventing the symptoms. Medication in conjunction with some form of psychotherapy has been found to be the most effective in helping a young person manage his or her symptoms (Andreescu, Mulsant, & Emanuel, 2008). Family therapies have been found helpful in managing the daily problems of having a child with bipolar disorder.

MEDICATION

Medication, in the form of a mood stabilizer, is the first line of treatment for bipolar disorder (Hirschfeld, 2005; Sachs, Printz, Kahn, Carpenter, & Docherty, 2000). Lithium was the first mood stabilizer approved by the U.S. Food and Drug Administration (FDA). Lithium is a very effective medication for stabilizing the mood changes in bipolar disorder. Additionally, antiseizure medications (also called anticonvulsants) commonly used to treat epilepsy and seizure disorders have been found effective for use as mood stabilizers. Two of the most commonly used antiseizure medications for treating bipolar disorder are Depakote and Tegretol.

A common theme discussed throughout this book is the controversy of treating children and adolescents with medications developed and tested on adults. Although there is controversy about using mood stabilizers to treat children with bipolar disorder, research on this class of medication has been conducted with children. Depakote, Tegretol, and lithium have all been studied and found to effectively treat bipolar disorder in children and adolescents (Hirschfeld, 2005; Sachs et al., 2000). In addition, Depakote has been approved by the FDA to treat seizure disorders in children as young as ten years old. Therefore, it may be less stigmatizing for a physician to treat a child with bipolar disorder with Depakote rather than lithium.

Treatments for bipolar disorder have improved over the last ten years, but everyone responds differently to medications, and all medications have side effects. Many of the serious side effects of a medication will affect a very small portion of those taking it; however, the chance of side effects always exists. Some medications used for treating bipolar disorder have been linked to serious problems; therefore, everyone taking them should be aware of the possible side effects, be monitored closely, and see a doctor regularly. Any problems with a medication should be immediately reported to the doctor.

Possible side effects of lithium include:

- Loss of coordination;
- Excessive thirst;
- Frequent urination;
- Blackouts;
- Seizures;
- Slurred speech;
- Fast, slow, irregular, or pounding heartbeat;
- Hallucinations (seeing things or hearing voices that do not exist);
- Changes in vision;
- Itching, rash;

- Swelling of the eyes, face, lips, tongue, throat, hands, feet, ankles, or lower legs;
- Problems with kidney and thyroid functioning.

Some possible side effects linked with Depakote include:

- Changes in weight
- Nausea
- Stomach pain
- Vomiting
- Anorexia
- Loss of appetite
- Damage to the liver or pancreas

In addition to the side effects listed above, Depakote has been found to increase levels of the male hormone testosterone in some females and to lead to a condition called polycystic ovarian syndrome (PCOS; Calabrese et al., 2005; Vainionpaa et al., 1999). Polycystic ovarian syndrome is a disease that can affect fertility and make the menstrual cycle become irregular. The symptoms of PCOS usually go away once a person stops taking Depakote. Pregnant females should not take Depakote because it has been linked to birth defects. Depakote, Tegretol, and other anticonvulsant medications come with an FDA warning. The warning states that anyone taking these medications should be closely monitored for new or worsening symptoms of depression, suicidal thoughts or behavior, or any unusual changes in mood or behavior.

Despite the possible side effects, children and teens with bipolar disorder can get better with these medications. Families must weigh the risk versus the benefits of having their children take one of these medications. Caregivers have complained that medications cause their child to experience changes in their personalities and to be out of it or spaced out. At the same time, persons taking mood stabilizers complain that the medications make them feel slowed down, unproductive, and not themselves. They are used to the mania or hypomania and they like it. Feeling *normal* does not feel normal to them. Because of this, it is not uncommon for persons to stop taking their medications in an effort to experience the high from mania, forgetting about the negative consequences that can result from poor decision making, risk taking, and other harmful behaviors. They also forget about the inevitable crash they will experience.

Each medication affects different people in different ways. Therefore, a psychiatrist may have to try out a couple of different medications before finding the most effective one for a particular person. In addition, antidepressant and/or antipsychotic medications are sometimes added to the medication regimen when a mood stabilizer is not enough to control depressive or psychotic symptoms (see chapter 5 for discussion of antidepressants and chapter 15 for antipsychotic medications). It is important to note that a person with bipolar disorder should never take an antidepressant without also taking a mood stabilizer. An antidepressant alone could result in a manic episode. It is also important to note that recent research through the National Institute of Mental Health (n.d.) is finding that adding an antidepressant to a mood stabilizer does not give any extra benefit. Research is ongoing.

PSYCHOSOCIAL INTERVENTIONS

There is limited research in the literature on evidence-based practices or programs designed specifically for youth with bipolar disorder. The majority of bipolar research focuses on adults. The limited existing research for youth experiencing bipolar disorder has focused on cognitive-behavioral therapy, family-focused therapy, interpersonal and social rhythm therapy, and psychoeducation. All of these interventions share many of the same practices. They also use many of the same practices discussed in other chapters for treating illnesses such as anxiety disorders, depression, or attention deficit hyperactivity disorder.

Family-Focused Therapy

Family-focused therapy (FFT) was first developed for adults diagnosed with bipolar disorder and their families and has since been adapted and is under evaluation for use with youth (Miklowitz & Goldstein, 1997; Miller, Solomon, Ryan, & Keitner, 2004; Simoneau, Miklowitz, Richards, Saleem, & George, 1999). It is considered an adjunct to medication and not a replacement for medication. Family-focused therapy is a time-limited treatment, lasting for approximately twenty-one sessions. Sessions initially occur weekly and then titrate down to occur twice a month and finally monthly. Each session presents the theoretical underpinnings that families need in order to understand and cope (psychoeducation) and the skills to improve family communication and problem solving (expressed emotion). As the focus of the first seven sessions of FFT, psychoeducation helps family members gain a better understanding of early onset bipolar disorder, what to expect with the illness, and available treatment options. Families learn to identify early warning signs of a manic or depressive episode so that they can intervene early, before the symptoms become worse. The remaining sessions focus on teaching the family new communication and problem-solving skills to enhance the overall quality of family interactions and to manage problems associated with the illness. The therapist teaches the family the new skills and the family practices the skills in sessions. The therapist provides feedback to the family during the practice sessions. Between sessions, the family is given a homework assignment to track the times they use or attempt to use the new skills at home. After treatment ends, booster sessions are sometimes used as a way to help the family maintain the new skills.

Interpersonal and Social Rhythm Therapy

Interpersonal and social rhythm therapy (IPSRT) is an evidence-based program (Frank, 2005). As with FFT, IPSRT is considered an adjunct to medication rather than a standalone treatment. It is a time-limited intervention focused on teaching youth skills to manage their illness and improve relationships. A key component of IPSRT is to develop and maintain a daily routine (social rhythm) that is based on individual biological and social rhythms, with specified times to sleep, do homework, and eat meals, for example. The theoretical underpinning of IPSRT is that maintaining a social rhythm will help protect against manic episodes. Therapists teach youth skills to manage stressful life events and to stay on track with their social rhythm; they also emphasize the importance of and techniques for adhering to the prescribed medication regime.

Cognitive-Behavioral Therapy

Cognitive-behavioral therapy (CBT) is the most extensively tested psychosocial treatment for depression. It is being used as an adjunct to medication for youth with bipolar disorder (Pavuluri et al., 2004). It has been found to be effective in treating both children and adolescents experiencing depression. The focus of CBT is to change how one thinks and acts as a means of improving depression.

This is based on the theory that depression is both caused and maintained by negative or irrational beliefs.

Cognitive-behavioral therapy is structured and time limited, lasting anywhere from six to twelve weeks. The first goal of CBT is to help youth realize that they can control their own behaviors and therefore can change the depression. The therapist works with the youth by teaching strategies to stop, confront, and change irrational and negative thought patterns.

Mood diaries or emotions charts are common tools used to assist young people to monitor thoughts, actions, physiological sensations, emotions, and events and to become aware of how these factors affect their depression. The therapist also teaches the youth problem-solving, coping, self-monitoring, relaxation, and social skills. Learning ways to relax in stressful situations helps the youth feel more competent and opens the door to trying out other skills. Homework is used as a strategy for increasing learning and integrating the skills being developed.

CASE STUDIES

Tina

Tina is the thirteen-year-old who always made good grades, had lots of friends, and loved sports. Her behavior suddenly changed. She began having trouble sleeping, often pacing around the house throughout the night. She was unable to sleep more than two hours a night for several days, but she claimed not to feel tired.

At times her mood changed very quickly from overly happy to angry and irritable. She cursed at others for no known reason. She started talking rapidly about a lot of different things, but mainly she boasted about how much smarter and more popular she was than everyone else. During school, her behaviors were very disruptive. She would talk over the teacher about things not related to the class.

Her parents became concerned that she was using drugs. They did not know how to handle the situation. The final straw for them was when she stole their car and went for a ride even though she was not old enough to drive. The police stopped her for speeding. When they learned that she was not old enough to drive, they took her to the juvenile detention center. Her parents were able to convince the judge to drop the charges and allow them to take her to a hospital for drug and alcohol treatment.

When Tina was taken in for treatment, the doctor ordered a toxicology screening to determine what drugs she had been taking. Tina denied using drugs or alcohol. Her toxicology report came back negative for drugs and alcohol. She was transferred to the psychiatric adolescent unit of the hospital, and with parental consent, was started on Depakote against her will. Her parents did not want her to take the medication, but they did not know what else to do. After spending three weeks in the hospital, Tina was discharged and returned home to her normal life and school. She was given a follow-up appointment with her psychiatrist.

A few days after leaving the hospital, Tina told her parents that she was feeling good and did not need to take the Depakote. She stopped taking it. After a few days, she began experiencing rapid cycling of her moods and was again hospitalized. She was discharged with the same follow-up plan as for her last discharge, but was strongly counseled about the importance of staying on her medications.

Jack

When Jack was seven years old, his parents noticed changes in his mood and behaviors over the course of several months. One minute, he would act silly and say silly things. He would make weird faces, laugh hysterically out of the clear blue, and run around the house. The next minute he would begin crying and tell his parents that he hated himself because he was ugly and stupid. He would apologize over and over for things that he perceived he did wrong, but in reality these things were of no consequence. He went through periods of not needing sleep and exhibiting extreme levels of energy. During these times, he would start an activity and then move on to another activity without finishing the first. At other times, he would isolate himself in his room and not show any interest in playing video games or playing with friends. He would hit his baby sister, punch a wall, or exhibit other unprovoked aggressive behaviors. He told his parents that he did these things because the voices were telling him to do bad things.

Jack's parents became frustrated with Jack's behavior, believing he was doing these things to get attention. Punishment did not seem to change his behaviors. One day, he choked his baby sister, bruising her neck. His mother called the police. The police said that they could not do anything to help because he was only seven years old. They told her to call social services because he was a danger to his sister. Social services helped the parents find a residential facility, where Jack was admitted for long-term care. After six months in the treatment facility, Jack was discharged to return home. His behaviors improved significantly while in the facility. Each day, nurses gave him his medication and ensured that he swallowed it. He reached the top level of the facility's behavioral program, which allowed him to be discharged and return home.

Questions for Review

1. What do these real life scenarios have in common?
2. What are the differences?
3. Now that you know what happened to each of the youths, do you have any different thoughts on how you would have handled the situation if you were the families' social worker?

REFERENCES

Andreescu, C., Mulsant, B. H., & Emanuel, J. E. (2008). Complementary and alternative medicine in the treatment of bipolar disorder: A review of the evidence. *Journal of Affective Disorders, 110*, 16.

Calabrese, J. R., Shelton, M. D., Rapport, D. J., Youngstrom, E. A., Jackson, K., Bilali, S., . . . Findling, R. L. (2005). A 20-month, double-blind, maintenance trial of lithium versus divalproex in rapid-cycling bipolar disorder. *American Journal of Psychiatry, 162*, 2152–2161.

Frank, E. (2005). *Treating bipolar disorder: A clinician's guide to interpersonal and social rhythm therapy.* New York: Guilford Press.

Hirschfeld, R. M. (2005). *Guideline watch: Practice guideline for the treatment of patients with bipolar disorder* (2nd ed.). Arlington, VA: American Psychiatric Association. Retrieved from http://psychiatryonline.org/pb/assets/raw/sitewide/practice _guidelines/guidelines/bipolar-watch.pdf

Miklowitz, D. J., & Goldstein, M. J. (1997). *Bipolar disorder: A family-focused treatment approach.* New York: Guilford Press.

Miller, I., Solomon, D. A., Ryan, C. E., & Keitner, G. I. (2004). Does adjunctive family therapy enhance recovery from bipolar I mood episodes? *Journal of Affective Disorders, 82*, 431–436.

National Institute of Mental Health. (n.d.). *Bipolar disorder.* Retrieved from www.nimh .nih.gov/health/topics/bipolar-disorder/index.shtml

Pavuluri, M. N., Graczyk, P. A., Henry, D. B., Carbray, J. A., Heidenrich, J., & Miklowitz, D. J. (2004). Child- and family-focused cognitive behavioral therapy for pediatric bipolar disorder: Development and preliminary results. *Journal of the American Academy of Child and Adolescent Psychiatry, 43,* 528–537.

Sachs, G. S., Printz, D. J., Kahn, D. A., Carpenter, D., & Docherty, J. P. (2000). *The Expert Consensus Guideline Series: Medication treatment of bipolar disorder 2000,* 1–104. New York: McGraw-Hill Healthcare Information Programs. Retrieved from http://www.senon-online.com/Documentation/telechargement/guidelines/guide lines%20TB%20Dep/Bipolar_2000.pdf

Simoneau, T. L., Miklowitz, D. J., Richards, J. A., Saleem, R., & George, E. L. (1999). Bipolar disorder and family communication: Effects of a psychoeducational treatment program. *Journal of Abnormal Psychology, 108,* 588–597.

Vainionpaa, L. K., Rattya, J., Knip, M., Tapanainen, J. S., Pakarinen, A. J., Lanning, P., . . . Isojarvi, J. I. (1999). Valproate-induced hyperandrogenism during pubertal maturation in girls with epilepsy. *Annals of Neurology, 45,* 444–450.

CHAPTER 14

Schizophrenia

SCHIZOPHRENIA IS A BRAIN DISORDER that results in
strange thinking, abnormal feelings, and odd behaviors. Persons with schizophrenia often interpret reality in abnormal
ways and have difficulty discerning real events from imaginary events. Because of this, untreated schizophrenia can
result in serious problems that interfere with all areas of
a person's life, resulting in outcomes such as poverty,
homelessness, legal problems, relationship difficulties, family conflicts, and inability to work. On television people with schizophrenia are often
depicted as homeless persons walking around
wearing too many layers of clothing and talking to themselves. Although this picture
may be true for a very small population of
people who are not receiving treatment,
many other people who receive treatment can experience relief from
their symptoms and lead full
happy lives. For others, coping with symptoms and

the ongoing need for intensive supports and services can be lifelong. Development of schizophrenia is very rare prior to adulthood; however, it does happen. Persons who develop schizophrenia in childhood or adolescence usually experience a more severe, chronic form of the disorder (Vyas & Gogtay, 2012).

CAUSES

Schizophrenia affects an estimated 1 percent of the population. Most of what we know about schizophrenia has come from studies with adults. The prevalence of the disorder is the same across genders, races, and ethnicities (Regier et al., 1993). The exact causes of schizophrenia are not completely known; however, much progress in understanding schizophrenia has been made through genetic and brain research. Years ago, ineffective mothering was thought to be the cause. Current research suggests that schizophrenia is caused by many factors, including genes, brain chemistry, and environmental factors.

GENES AND SCHIZOPHRENIA

Researchers believe that genetics plays a role in the development of schizophrenia (Harrison & Weinberger, 2005). Although schizophrenia affects 1 percent of the general population, the risk increases to 10 percent for persons who have a parent or sibling with schizophrenia (Cannon et al, 2008; Regier et al., 1993). The highest risk of heritability (genetics) for schizophrenia occurs with identical twins (Cardno & Gottesman, 2000; Masi, Mucci, & Pari, 2006; Nicolson et al., 2000). When an identical twin develops schizophrenia, the other twin has an increased risk as high as 40 to 65 percent of also developing it. Adoption studies have helped inform scientists on the causes. Adopted children with a biological parent with schizophrenia have a higher risk of developing psychosis whether or not they lived with the biological parent. If one of their adoptive parents, rather than a biological parent, has schizophrenia, they are at no more risk than the general population. Researchers have linked high levels of genetic mutations involving multiple genes and genetic malfunctioning that affects development of higher level brain functioning to schizophrenia (Walsh et al., 2008). Many research studies on the genetic connections to schizophrenia continue.

SCHIZOPHRENIA AND THE BRAIN

Scientists do not believe that genetics alone causes schizophrenia (Mueser & McGurk, 2004). Research findings suggest that other factors in addition to genetic predisposition are the contributors. Prenatal insults to the brain that result in changes to brain structure and chemistry are being studied as possible contributors to schizophrenia (Mueser & McGurk, 2004). Prenatal insults may include viral infections, lack of oxygen at birth, starvation, or an untreated blood type incompatibility between a mother and fetus. There have also been studies that have found changes to the dopamine and glutamine neurotransmitters in persons with schizophrenia (Sedvall & Farde, 1995; Seeman, Hong-Chang, & Hubert, 1993).

Other studies have shown differences in the size of ventricles in the brain and differences in the activity of grey matter. Brain scans have shown that children who experience psychotic symptoms prior to puberty exhibit progressively abnormal brain development (Giedd et al., 1999; Rapoport et al., 1999; Thompson et al., 2001).

Researchers at the National Institute of Mental Health (NIMH) have been studying the brains of children with early onset schizophrenia using high-resolution MRI scans (Giedd et al., 1999). The children in the study are evaluated by the researchers every two years. The researchers hypothesize that an insult to the back of a child's brain contributes to the onset of schizophrenia. As they have followed children through the years, they have found evidence of significant shrinkage in brain tissue volume that starts in the back of the brain. The brain tissue continues to shrink as the disease progresses. These same researchers have found that healthy siblings of youth with schizophrenia show similar thinning, but this abnormality goes away as they age. Researchers have also found that the brains of children with schizophrenia share the same abnormalities as those of adults with schizophrenia (Gogtay et al., 2008). Home movies taken during childhood show that persons with adult-onset schizophrenia experienced uneven motor development in childhood, such as unusual crawling as children. This lends support to the idea that they may have had abnormalities in brain functioning during childhood, but the symptoms of schizophrenia did not become evident until they reached adulthood. Because a child's brain is constantly changing, it may take years before the effects of the brain insult are evident.

SIGNS AND SYMPTOMS

The age of onset and the developmental level of a person will affect how symptoms are experienced and responsiveness to treatment. Research suggests that persons who experience childhood onset of schizophrenia will have a different presentation of symptoms than those who experience onset as adults and adolescents. Children with schizophrenia may be even more seriously impaired. They are also more anxious and disruptive than patients with adult-onset schizophrenia were as children. However, the classifications of symptoms are the same regardless of age of onset. The symptoms of schizophrenia are classified as positive, negative, and cognitive (*DSM-5*; American Psychiatric Association, 2013).

Positive Symptoms

Positive symptoms are thoughts, behaviors, or sensory perceptions experienced by a person with a mental illness that are not experienced by other persons. They are an exaggeration or a distortion of a person's normal functioning. Positive symptoms include hallucinations, delusions, thought disorders, and movement disorders. Psychotic symptoms usually appear later in the disease, most often between the ages of sixteen and thirty. Males tend to experience symptoms at an earlier age than females.

Hallucinations are distortions of reality that may come in the form of hearing, seeing, smelling, tasting, or feeling something that is not real; however, these sensations feel real to the person experiencing them. Hearing things that are not there (auditory hallucinations) is the most common type of hallucination. When someone experiences an auditory hallucination, he or she may hear voices or other sounds. Some people experience voices that say negative or demeaning things such as "you are a bad person" or "you cannot do anything right." Command hallucinations are experienced as one or more voices telling the person to do something such as "hit your sister" or "burn down the house." Because the voices are real to the person experiencing them, he or she may feel compelled to do what they say to do.

Delusions are beliefs in something that is not true. They are false beliefs about something, such as believing that the government is monitoring one's thoughts or controlling one's behavior. They can also cause a person to believe that he or she is someone or something else, such as a member of royalty or the most intelligent person in the world.

Thought disorders appear in the form of unusual ways of thinking. The person's thoughts may be disorganized and result in stopping speech in mid-sentence. It is not uncommon for someone experiencing a thought disorder to make up words or to take a long time to respond to a question.

Negative Symptoms

Negative symptoms are thoughts, behaviors, or sensory perceptions experienced by the general population that are not experienced by a person with a mental illness. They disrupt a person's normal emotions or behaviors. For example, a person may neglect personal hygiene such as brushing teeth, taking baths, or changing into clean clothes. Isolation and disinterest in relationships often occur. Lacking motivation to do things, such as go to school or work, is also common. Negative symptoms may appear to be laziness, which can cause frustration in people who do not understand that these are symptoms of schizophrenia. The majority of antipsychotic medications do not treat the negative symptoms.

Cognitive Symptoms

Cognitive symptoms interfere with thought processes, resulting in problems understanding and using information. It is thought that a person with schizophrenia is born with the cognitive symptoms. If that is the case, a person will show signs of cognitive problems from the beginning of life, but may not develop negative or positive symptoms until later in life. The ability to do well in school and other areas of life will be disrupted for these children because they cannot make sense of information and have trouble paying attention and remembering things. These symptoms are often attributed to other conditions, resulting in the lack of appropriate treatment.

DIAGNOSING SCHIZOPHRENIA

Diagnosing schizophrenia can be difficult, particularly in young children and for someone who does not have experience in pediatric psychiatry. The first step in diagnosing schizophrenia should be a complete physical that includes toxicology screening and brain scans to rule out other possible explanations such as a medical condition or substance abuse. Once physical health problems and drug and alcohol abuse have been ruled out, a complete psychosocial history should be completed to investigate the onset of the youth's problems and the family's history of health/mental health problems, followed by a functional assessment of the youth to evaluate cognitive skills and daily functioning and a review of the youth's functioning at school.

In the *DSM-IV* (American Psychiatric Association, 1994), a diagnosis of schizophrenia required continuous signs of schizophrenia to have been present for at least six months, with at least two symptoms (positive, negative, and/or cognitive) lasting for at least one month. The severity of the symptoms must cause serious impairment in a person's ability to function. The core of the diagnostic criteria for schizophrenia in the *DSM-IV* remains the same in the *DSM-5*; however, there are some minor and some significant differences.

In the *DSM-5*, the number of symptoms was changed so that a person needs at least one positive symptom: hallucinations, delusions, or disorganized language. A significant change from the *DSM-IV* to the *DSM-5* is the elimination of subtypes of schizophrenia. The *DSM-IV* classified the subtypes as paranoid, disorganized, catatonic, undifferentiated, and residual. A person was diagnosed with a subtype based on the symptoms he or she was experiencing prominently. The *DSM-IV* characterized the paranoid schizophrenia subtype by hallucinations and delusions that follow persecutory and/or grandiose themes. The disorganized subtype involved severe functional impairment. Characteristic symptoms of this subtype included disorganized thinking and behavior. The catatonic subtype was characterized by psychomotor disturbance in the form of complete immobility and lack of responsiveness, bizarre posturing, or excessive movement. The undifferentiated subtype was characterized by psychosis and the negative symptoms of schizophrenia, such as lack of interest in social interactions or flat affect, but not by any other criteria for any of the other types. Finally, the residual subtype was characterized by at least one episode of one of the other four subtypes of schizophrenia and negative symptoms, but no prominent positive symptoms of the disease. These subtypes are not included in the *DSM-5* because they were not found helpful in determining treatment and they lack reliability and validity (Helmes & Landmark, 2003; Linscott, Allardyce, & van Os, 2010; Tandon & Maj, 2008; Xu, 2011). Diagnosing schizophrenia has moved from categorizing symptoms as a subtype to a focus on measuring the severity of the dimensions of the disorder in each individual (Kupfer & Regier, 2011).

SCHIZOPHRENIA IN CHILDREN AND ADOLESCENTS

Onset of schizophrenia in youth under the age of fifteen is rare, affecting about 1 in 40,000 children (Masi et al., 2006). When it does occur, it can be difficult to recognize because it is so rare and because it emerges more slowly in children. Children normally do not experience a sudden onset of psychotic symptoms. The onset of symptoms is much slower. Research has shown that the earlier a person develops schizophrenia, the more severe the form of schizophrenia and the poorer the prognosis (Driver, Gogtay, & Rapoport, 2013). Prior to children experiencing psychosis, they often experience lags in motor and speech language development and a decline in full-scale IQ. This phase of the disease is called the *prodromal phase*. These developmental disturbances result in the child having difficulties in school and social situations and at home, but the lack of the psychotic symptoms makes it difficult to diagnose schizophrenia.

As the disease progresses, marked behavioral changes occur. Children may start talking about fears and ideas that are strange, saying things that do not make sense, clinging to parents, or seeming to withdraw and appear to be in their own world. They often have trouble discriminating between their dreams and reality or may confuse television or movies with reality. They often experience a loss of social skills and self-help skills. They become withdrawn and lose interest in having friends or being social. Children with schizophrenia are often mistakenly thought to have a pervasive developmental disorder (PDD) such as autism or Asperger's syndrome. About a third of children with schizophrenia have transient symptoms of PDD, such as rocking, posturing, and arm flapping, and like children with PDD, they experience impairment across all life domains. Although diagnosing schizophrenia is difficult due to the similarity of its symptoms to those of PDD, the disorders can be distinguished. Autism develops earlier in children. It is usually diagnosed by the time a child turns three, whereas schizophrenia tends to develop when a child is six or seven years old. Unlike a child with autism, a child with schizophrenia will experience hallucinations or delusions that persist for at least six months.

VIOLENCE

The majority of persons with schizophrenia are not violent toward other persons (Swanson et al., 2006; Walsh, Buchanan, & Fahy, 2002). However, there is a prevailing belief that persons with schizophrenia are often violent. This is mostly due to the media. In television shows or movies, persons with schizophrenia are portrayed as violent and unpredictable. The news media does not provide information about the majority of persons with schizophrenia who are doing well in life and those who have never been violent. Instead, it focuses on the very small minority of instances in which something tragic occurs. If a person with schizophrenia does become violent or dangerous, violence is usually directed toward a family member and most often occurs as a result of psychosis. For instance, Mary believed an alien had invaded her mother's body and was out to harm her. Mary attacked her mother in an attempt to protect herself from the alien. Again, these instances are very rare. Persons with schizophrenia are more likely to harm themselves than to harm someone else. An estimated 10 percent of persons with schizophrenia commit suicide.

TOOLS FOR ASSESSING THE SYMPTOMS OF SCHIZOPHRENIA

There are some useful tools for measuring the positive and negative symptoms of schizophrenia. These instruments measure the severity of symptoms and help monitor the effectiveness of treatment.

The Positive and Negative Syndrome Scale

The Positive and Negative Syndrome Scale (PANSS; Kay, Fiszbein, & Opler, 1987) is probably the most well known and utilized assessment tool for monitoring treatment effectiveness for schizophrenia. The PANSS is an easy to administer and highly reliable tool for measuring the symptoms of schizophrenia. It consists of thirty items that are rated on a seven-point Likert scale whereby a score of *1* means symptoms are absent and a score of *7* means that symptoms are extreme. Of the thirty items, seven measure negative symptoms (PANSS-N). The remaining twenty-three items measure positive symptoms (PANSS-P).

The Four-Item Positive Symptoms Rating Scale and Brief Negative Symptom Assessment

The four-item Positive Symptoms Rating Scale (PSRS) and Brief Negative Symptom Assessment (BNSA) measure levels of positive and negative symptoms associated with schizophrenia (Alphs, Morlock, Coon, Van Willigenburg, &

Panagides, 2010). Each of these instruments consists of four items. The PSRS is measured on a seven-point Likert scale. As with the PANSS, a score of *1* means that the symptom is not present and a score of *7* means that the symptoms are severe. The BNSA is measured on a six-point Likert scale with a score of *1* meaning that the symptoms are not present and a *6* meaning that the symptoms are severe. Positive symptoms measured include hallucinations, suspiciousness, unusual thought content, and conceptual disorganization. Negative symptoms measured by the BNSA include slow response time, blunted affect, reduced social drive, and poor hygiene.

Scale for the Assessment of Negative Symptoms

The Scale for the Assessment of Negative Symptoms (SANS; Andreasen, 1982, 1989) is a measurement instrument used in the field to assess the negative symptoms. The SANS assesses across five areas of negative symptoms: affective blunting, impoverished thinking and cognition (alogia), lack of energy (avolition), disturbance of attention, and lack of interest or pleasure (anhedonia). The SANS is conducted on a six-point scale with *0* meaning that there are no negative symptoms and *5* indicating a severe level of the negative symptom.

CASE STUDIES

Gus

Gus is a ten-year-old admitted to a psychiatric hospital after exhibiting aggressive behaviors at home and school. At school, Gus refused to stay in his seat and complete his work. When confronted by the teacher, he kicked over his desk and ran out of the school. He was picked up by police a few blocks away from the school and taken home. After the police left, Gus's behavior escalated. He destroyed his room. When his mother tried to calm him down, he ran into the kitchen, grabbed a large knife, and threatened to stab himself in the neck. His father restrained him and took the knife away. His parents drove him to the hospital, where he was evaluated by a psychiatrist. During the interview, Gus told the psychiatrist that he was seeing scary people. The psychiatrist admitted Gus to the children's unit for observation.

During his first few days on the unit, Gus was restrained and secluded multiple times for throwing chairs and doing other things that were threatening to other patients and staff. The psychiatrist started him on medications. The medications made Gus very drowsy. He spent many hours sleeping each day. After spending a week in the hospital, Gus was discharged to return home. He was given a follow-up appointment with another psychiatrist and returned to school.

Consider the following questions:

1. What symptoms was Gus experiencing?

2. Does he meet the criteria for schizophrenia? Explain. If he does, which type?

3. Based on your current knowledge, what interventions would you suggest? Do you believe that the appropriate intervention or treatment was provided?

4. Who should be included in the treatment planning and interventions?

5. What barriers might get in the way of effectively intervening?

6. What suggestions/thoughts/ideas do you have for his family?

Erin

Erin is a seventeen-year-old in her junior year of high school. She was always an A student and very active in student government. She was the vice president of her class. Midway through her junior year, Erin suddenly stopped hanging out with friends. Her grades declined rapidly. Whereas she had always been very particular about wearing the latest fashions and would never leave the house without makeup, she began wearing sweats to school, and she stopped wearing makeup and attending to her personal hygiene, such as washing her hair. She said things to her parents that were very odd and sometimes started giggling for no reason. Her parents suspected that she was using drugs. She became very angry at her parents when they questioned her about the changes.

A few weeks after there were notable changes in Erin's behavior, the school counselor, who was very concerned, contacted Erin's parents. Erin had turned in a test that had rambling sentences scribbled all over the page and had not answered the test questions. Her parents picked her up and took her to the hospital. A full medical evaluation was completed, including screening for drugs and alcohol. Nothing turned up. Her parents were questioned about any family history of mental illness. They both said there was no family history of mental illness.

Erin was admitted to the psychiatric unit of the hospital and was started on a regimen of antipsychotic medications. After a few weeks in the hospital, Erin did not show any improvement in her symptoms. She denied that anything was wrong and screamed at her parents to take her home.

How would you answer the following questions?

1. What symptoms was Erin experiencing?
2. Does she meet the criteria for schizophrenia? Explain. If she does, which type?
3. Based on your current knowledge, what interventions would you suggest? Do you believe that the appropriate intervention or treatment was provided?
4. Who should be included in the treatment planning and interventions?
5. What barriers might get in the way of effectively intervening?
6. What suggestions/thoughts/ideas do you have for her family?

REFERENCES

Alphs, L., Morlock, R., Coon, C., Van Willigenburg, A., & Panagides, J. (2010). The 4-Item Negative Symptom Assessment (NSA-4) Instrument: A simple tool for evaluating negative symptoms in schizophrenia following brief training. *Psychiatry, 7*(7), 26–32.

American Psychiatric Association. (1994). *Diagnostic and statistical manual of mental disorders* (4th ed.). Washington, DC: Author.

American Psychiatric Association. (2013). *Diagnostic and statistical manual of mental disorders* (5th ed.). Washington, DC: Author.

Andreasen, N. C. (1982). Negative symptoms in schizophrenia: Definition and reliability. *Archives of General Psychiatry, 39*, 784–788.

Andreasen, N. C. (1989). The scale for the assessment of negative symptoms (SANS): Conceptual and theoretical foundations. *British Journal of Psychiatry Supplements, 7*, 49–58.

Cannon, T. D., Cadenhead, K., Cornblatt, B., Woods, S. W., Addington, J., Walker, E., . . . Heinssen, R. (2008). Prediction of psychosis in high-risk youth: A multi-site longitudinal study in North America. *Archives of General Psychiatry, 65*, 28–37.

Cardno, A. G., & Gottesman, I. I. (2000). Twin studies of schizophrenia: From bow-and-arrow concordances to Star Wars Mx and functional genomics. *American Journal of Medical Genetics, 97*, 12–17.

Driver, D. I., Gogtay, N., & Rapoport, J. L. (2013). Childhood onset schizophrenia and early onset schizophrenia spectrum disorders. *Child and Adolescent Psychiatric Clinics of North America, 22*, 539–555. doi:10.1016/j.chc.2013.04.001

Giedd, J. N., Blumenthal, J., Jeffries, N. O., Castellanos, F. X., Liu, H., Zijdenbos, A., . . . Rapoport, J. L. (1999). Brain development during childhood and adolescence: A longitudinal MRI study. *Nature Neuroscience, 2*, 861–863.

Gogtay, N., Lu, A., Leow, A. D., Klunder, A. D., Lee, A. D., Chavez, A., . . . Thompson, P. M. (2008). Three-dimensional brain growth abnormalities in childhood-onset schizophrenia visualized by using tensor-based morphometry. *Proceedings of the National Academy of Sciences of the United States of America, 105*(41), 15979–15984.

Harrison, P. J., & Weinberger, D. R. (2005). Schizophrenia genes, gene expression, and neuropathology: On the matter of their convergence. *Molecular Psychiatry, 10*, 40–68.

Helmes, E., & Landmark, J. (2003). Subtypes of schizophrenia: A cluster analytic approach. *Canadian Journal of Psychiatry, 48*, 702–708.

Kay, S. R., Fiszbein, A., & Opler, L. A. (1987). The positive and negative syndrome scale (PANSS) for schizophrenia. *Schizophrenia Bulletin, 13*, 261–276.

Kupfer, D. J., & Regier, D. A. (2011). Neuroscience, clinical evidence, and the future of psychiatric classification in DSM-5. *American Journal of Psychiatry, 68*, 672–674.

Linscott, R. J., Allardyce, J., & van Os, J. (2010). Seeking verisimilitude in a class: A systematic review of evidence that the criterial clinical symptoms of schizophrenia are taxonic. *Schizophrenia Bulletin, 36*, 811–829.

Masi, G., Mucci, M., & Pari, C. (2006). Children with schizophrenia: Clinical picture and pharmacological treatment. *CNS Drugs, 20*, 841–866.

Mueser, K., & McGurk, S. (2004). Schizophrenia. *The Lancet, 363*, 2063–2072.

Nicolson, R., Lenane, M., Hamburger, S. D., Fernandez, T., Bedwell, J., & Rapoport, J. L. (2000). Lessons from childhood-onset schizophrenia. *Brain Research Review, 31*(2–3), 147–156.

Rapoport, J. L., Giedd, J. N., Blumenthal, J., Hamburger, S., Jeffries, N., Fernandez, T., . . . Evans, A. (1999). Progressive cortical change during adolescence in childhood-onset schizophrenia: A longitudinal magnetic resonance imaging study. *Archives of General Psychiatry, 56*, 649–654.

Regier, D. A., Narrow, W. E., Rae, D. S., Manderscheid, R. W., Locke, B. Z., & Goodwin, F. K. (1993). The de facto US mental and addictive disorders service system: Epidemiologic catchment area prospective 1-year prevalence rates of disorders and services. *Archives of General Psychiatry, 50*, 85–94.

Sedvall, G., & Farde, L. (1995). Chemical brain anatomy in schizophrenia. *The Lancet*, *346*, 743–749.

Seeman, P., Hong-Chang, G., & Hubert, V. T. (1993). Dopamine D4 receptors elevated in schizophrenia. *Nature, 365*, 441–445.

Swanson, J. W., Swartz, M. S., Van Dorn, R. A., Elbogen, E., Wager, H. R., Rosenheck, R. A., . . . Lieberman, J. A. (2006). A national study of violent behavior in persons with schizophrenia. *Archives of General Psychiatry, 63*, 490–499.

Tandon, R., & Maj, M. (2008). Nosological status and definition of schizophrenia: Some considerations for DSM-V and ICD-11. *Asian Journal of Psychiatry, 1*, 22–27.

Thompson, P. M., Vidal, C., Giedd, J. N., Gochman, P., Blumenthal, J., Nicolson, R., . . . Rapoport, J. L. (2001). Mapping adolescent brain change reveals dynamic wave of accelerated gray matter loss in very early-onset schizophrenia. *Proceedings of the National Academy of Sciences of the United States of America, 98*(20), 11650–11655.

Vyas, N. S., & Gogtay, N. (2012). Treatment of early onset schizophrenia: Recent trends, challenges and future considerations. *Frontiers in Psychiatry, 3*. doi:10.3389/fpsyt.2012.00029.

Walsh, E., Buchanan, A., & Fahy, T. (2002). Violence and schizophrenia: Examining the evidence. *British Journal of Psychiatry, 180*, 490–495.

Walsh, T., McClellan, J. M., McCarthy, S. E., Addington, A. M., Pierce, S. B., Cooper, G. M., . . . Sebat, J. (2008). Rare structural variants disrupt multiple genes in neuro-developmental pathways in schizophrenia. *Science, 320*(5875), 539–543.

Xu, T. Y. (2011). The subtypes of schizophrenia. *Shanghai Archives of Psychiatry, 23*, 106–108. Retrieved from http://www.shanghaiarchivesofpsychiatry.org/assets/15-shanghaiarchivesofpsychiatry-april2011-pgs106-107-forumsubtypes schizophrenia.pdf

CHAPTER 15

Treatment of Schizophrenia

CURRENTLY, there is no cure for schizophrenia, but hope exists in the research community that a cure will be discovered within the next decade. Additionally, it is predicted that schizophrenia can be prevented in persons with high risk factors through further understanding of genes and brain chemistry. Unfortunately, we are not there yet. There is currently no sure way to prevent schizophrenia. However, people who possess risk factors for schizophrenia can minimize their symptoms or prevent them from getting worse by taking preventative measures such as reducing stress, getting adequate sleep, and avoiding drugs and alcohol. If symptoms do appear, early treatment may lessen the severity of the symptoms and improve the trajectory of the disorder.

There has been a shift in the understanding of the trajectory of schizophrenia—from the belief that a person with schizophrenia will live with the symptoms for life to a focus on remission and recovery from the symptoms of schizophrenia (see, for example, Emsley, Chiliza, Asmal, & Lehloenya, 2011; Liberman, Kopelowicz, Ventura, & Gutkind, 2002). Recovery has varying meanings in the literature. The term *remission* implies that a person is experiencing minimal or no positive, negative, or cognitive problems. The term *recovery* has been described as not only a significant remission of symptoms, but also the ability to function in society, both socially and vocationally (Liberman et al., 2002).

Studies evaluating the concepts of remission and recovery have varied widely in their findings, with anywhere from 17 to 88 percent of persons experiencing remission (Andreasen et al., 2005; De Hert et al., 2007; Emsley et al., 2011). The overall findings of these studies suggest that the differences between those who experience recovery and those who do not are based on the level of functioning prior to the onset of the illness, age of onset, proximity between first sign of symptoms and treatment, and gender. Thus, persons who experienced remission or recovery are those who had higher functioning prior to onset of the illness, onset of the disease after age thirty, and treatment proximate to onset of symptoms; they were more likely to be female (Lambert, Karow, Leucht, Schimmelmann, & Naber, 2010). Those who experience early onset schizophrenia are much less likely to achieve recovery than those with later onset. Most persons with schizophrenia will have to cope with these symptoms throughout life. Psychosocial interventions can help a family cope with the illness and help youth with activities of daily functioning, but are not a substitute for medications.

An example of someone who experienced remission of symptoms and recovery to prior functioning is a young man diagnosed with schizophrenia who experienced his first psychotic episode in his mid-twenties. Prior to experiencing symptoms, he had a successful job, a girlfriend, and a close relationship with his parents. He experienced delusions that his parents were involved in the Oklahoma City bombing. He stayed in his room for days, making intricate maps and noting the ways that he believed his family was involved. He hardly slept and refused to eat. At the instigation of his family, he was committed to a hospital and required by court order to take medication. Several days after starting on the medication, he began questioning his thoughts, but he continued to believe them. After a few weeks on medication, he reported not knowing why he believed something so odd. He was discharged from the hospital and returned home to his family and his job.

MEDICATION

Treatment for childhood schizophrenia is mostly based on research conducted with adults (Masi, Mucci, & Pari, 2006). Antipsychotic medication is considered the first line of treatment. It can take as long as six months for a person to receive the full effects of antipsychotic medications (Lieberman et al., 2005). The positive symptoms often go away within days of starting the medication. Other symptoms, particularly the negative symptoms, take far longer.

Since the 1950s, antipsychotic medications have vastly improved. Older (typical) medications such as Haldol and Prolixin are used with decreasing frequency today. These older antipsychotics are effective in reducing hallucinations and delusions; however, they are not effective in treating the negative symptoms and they can cause debilitating side effects such as tardive dyskinesia (involuntary muscle movements) or muscle rigidity, spasms, tremors, and restlessness. These side effects, called *extrapyramidal side effects*, can become permanent.

The older antipsychotic medications have been mostly replaced by what are called new generation medications (atypical antipsychotics) such as Clozaril, Risperdol, Zyprexa, Seroquel, Geodon, Abilify, and Inverga. The older medications are far less expensive than the new generation medications. However, the new atypical antipsychotics do not pose as significant a threat for causing the extrapyramidal side effects as the older antipsychotics. On the other hand, like most medications, these new generation medicines come with their own set of side effects. Common side effects of atypical medications include weight gain, diabetes, and high cholesterol. It is estimated that as many as 62 percent of people with schizophrenia are overweight or obese, putting them at a high risk for cardiovascular morbidity and mortality (Ucok & Gaebel, 2008). In addition, persons with schizophrenia experience type II diabetes at nearly twice the rate of the general population.

The side effects of even the new generation medications can be scary. However, they are the first line of treatment and their benefits must be weighed against their risks. There can be great benefit from the atypical medications. These newer medications are more effective in treating the psychotic symptoms (positive symptoms) than the older medications. They also treat the negative symptoms. Additionally, some of the atypical medications appear to be effective in improving depressive symptoms, memory, and mental functioning and reducing aggression and suicidal ideation. These new generation antipsychotic medications have contributed greatly to the focus in the literature on remission and recovery. Each medication works in the brain a little differently from the others. Different people respond to each of the medications differently. Often this can result in what seems to families like trial and error to determine which medication will be most effective for an individual. Studies are currently underway to determine which of the atypical medications is most effective in treating specific symptoms.

It is also important for persons to follow their medication plan and not stop taking their medication without a psychiatrist's direction. The side effects of the new generation medications are often related to medication discontinuation. One factor consistent with all such medications is that every time a person discontinues medication without a doctor's advice, it becomes more difficult for him or her to get back to the level of functioning he or she had achieved before stopping (Andreasen, Liu, Ziebell, Vora, & Ho, 2013). Because of the side effects and the way that the psychotropic medications make them feel, people do not want to take these medications. It is not uncommon for people to *cheek* their medicine, meaning that they hold it between their gums and cheek and pretend to take it, but instead spit it out when no one is looking.

PSYCHOSOCIAL INTERVENTIONS

Currently, the National Registry of Evidence-based Practices and Programs established by the Substance Abuse and Mental Health Services Administration (SAMHSA; 2014) does not identify any evidence-based treatments specifically intended for early onset schizophrenia. Some of the interventions designed for adults with schizophrenia and some of the interventions designed for treatment of other mental health problems in youth have been adapted to treat childhood schizophrenia (Burns & Hoagwood, 2002; Burns, Hoagwood, & Mrazek, 1999). As described in chapter 2, wraparound is considered a promising practice for supporting and improving the lives of youth experiencing severe emotional or behavioral problems and their caregivers. Wraparound is not a specific treatment for schizophrenia; however, its focus on each family's individual needs, strengths, and desires can be an effective model for working with children diagnosed with schizophrenia and their families. Through the incorporation of formal (including evidence-based practices and programs) and informal services and community supports, families can receive the support and strength they need.

Although medication treats the symptoms, it does not help the youth and family with the day-to-day struggles of dealing with schizophrenia. Other psychosocial interventions are needed to help cope with the disease. Supportive therapies in conjunction with medication can be helpful in improving activities of daily living such as money management, grooming, and social adjustment and in supporting the caregivers. Psychosocial education teaches the youth, caregivers, and other family members about schizophrenia, its trajectory, and available treatments. Through education, families can learn to identify the early signs of problems so that they can seek help before symptoms exacerbate. Education can also help families understand the importance of medication and the detrimental effects of discontinuing a medication without psychiatrist supervision or the effects of not taking medication as prescribed. Families can also learn to watch for side effects that need attention from the psychiatrist.

Cognitive-Behavioral Therapy

Cognitive-behavioral therapy (CBT), in conjunction with medication, has been found to be helpful in teaching needed skills such as problem solving and stress reduction to help persons cope with their illnesses (Hogarty et al., 2002). Training in social skills and daily living skills can help youth to function better in school and participate in daily activities. Research has found that persons with early onset schizophrenia experience high levels of impairment in attaining educational or occupational goals and financial independence as adults.

Multisystemic Therapy-Psychiatric

Multisystemic therapy-psychiatric (MST-P) is an adaptation of the traditional multisystemic therapy model discussed in chapter 11 (Henggeler et al., 1999; Henggeler, Schoenwald, Rowland, & Cunningham, 2002; Rowland & Westlake, 2006). Multisystemic therapy-psychiatric is on SAMHSA's National Registry of Evidence-based Practices and Programs for the treatment of youth with behavioral and mental health problems. The goal of MST-P is to keep children who are at risk of psychiatric hospitalization in their home and community. Like traditional MST, MST-P utilizes a social ecological approach, focusing treatment on the youth, caregivers, school, or other environments contributing to problems; however, it has been adapted to specifically treat youth with serious behavioral and mental health problems rather than juvenile offenders. Multisystemic therapy-psychiatric integrates evidence-based psychiatric interventions into the MST model.

The MST-P team is slightly different from the traditional clinical MST team. It includes a part-time psychiatrist and a crisis caseworker in addition to the full-time doctoral level supervisor and four master's level therapists. The therapists receive specialized mental health training in addition to the five-day MST training. Rather than being the sole provider of treatment, they coordinate with the psychiatrist. Multisystemic treatment consultation is provided by both an MST expert consultant and an MST expert psychiatrist.

CASE STUDIES

Gus

Gus is the ten-year-old who was admitted to a psychiatric hospital after exhibiting aggressive behaviors at home and school. While in the hospital he was restrained and secluded multiple times for verbally and physically aggressive behaviors. He complained of seeing scary people. The psychiatrist diagnosed him with psychotic disorder not otherwise specified because Gus did not meet the criteria for a diagnosis of schizophrenia. The psychiatrist started Gus on antipsychotic medications. The medications made Gus very drowsy. He spent many hours sleeping each day. After spending a week in the hospital, he was discharged to return home. He was given a follow-up appointment with another psychiatrist and returned to school.

Gus could not keep his eyes open. He slept for hours. When awake, he seemed very drowsy and not completely coherent. He was not aggressive, but he also could not function. His mother took him to his psychiatric appointment. Unlike the psychiatrist who treated Gus in the hospital, this psychiatrist ordered a full medical evaluation and completed an in-depth psychosocial evaluation. During the interview, Gus disclosed that he was being sexually abused by a teenage neighbor. The psychiatrist took Gus off of the antipsychotic medication, started him on Paxil to help with anxiety, and referred him to a therapist who specialized in working with abused children. After six months, Gus was doing well in school and at home.

Erin

Erin is the seventeen-year-old who experienced serious changes in school functioning, peer relationships, and personal hygiene and began exhibiting odd behaviors such as giggling for no known reason. The school counselor contacted Erin's parents because Erin turned in a test that had rambling sentences scribbled all over the page and had not answered the test questions. Her parents picked her up and took her to the hospital. A full medical evaluation was completed. Screening for drugs and alcohol was negative.

Erin was admitted to the psychiatric unit of the hospital. After completing an in-depth psychiatric evaluation, the psychiatrist determined that Erin was hearing voices. Because Erin had not been having symptoms for at least six months, she diagnosed Erin with schizophreniform. The symptoms for schizophreniform are the same as those for schizophrenia, but there is no requirement for six months of symptoms. Erin was started on an antipsychotic medication. After a few weeks in the hospital, she was still not experiencing any improvement in symptoms. The psychiatrist was concerned that Erin was not improving. She began to suspect that Erin was not taking her medications. She asked the nurse to watch Erin swallow the pills and to check her mouth to be sure that she had swallowed them. After a few days, Erin's behaviors improved. She maintained an odd affect, but she denied hearing voices. Erin was discharged to her home after spending a month in the hospital.

Erin was not able to function in the classroom. She was referred to the school psychologist for testing. The psychologist recommended that Erin be considered to have an emotional disturbance and transferred to a special education class with other youth with emotional or behavioral problems. A meeting was held among Erin, her parents, the school counselor, the psychologist, a special education teacher, and her current teachers. Everyone but Erin agreed that she should be transferred to special education.

A few weeks after being discharged from the hospital, Erin's symptoms returned. She had stopped taking her medications. Her parents could not control her. She was taken back to the hospital. The doctor felt that Erin needed long-term care so Erin was transferred to the state psychiatric hospital, where she stayed for nearly three months. When she was discharged to her home, Erin never returned to school. She continued to go off and on her medications and was rehospitalized several times. She was diagnosed with schizophrenia and referred to the local community health center so that she could receive case management services in addition to psychiatrist services. The case manager helped Erin apply for Social Security Disability Insurance so that she could get disability checks to help support her and so that she could qualify for Medicaid. Erin continued to live with her parents.

What do these real life scenarios have in common? What are the differences? After learning what happened to each of the youths, do you have any different thoughts on how you would have handled the situation if you were the families' social worker?

REFERENCES

Andreasen, N. C., Carpenter, W. T., Jr., Kane, J. M., Lasser, R. A., Marder, S. R., & Weinberger, D. R. (2005). Remission in schizophrenia: Proposed criteria and rationale for consensus. *American Journal of Psychiatry*, *162*, 441–449.

Andreasen, N. C., Liu, D., Ziebell, S., Vora, A., & Ho, B. C. (2013). Relapse duration, treatment intensity, and brain tissue loss in schizophrenia: A prospective longitudinal MRI study. *American Journal of Psychiatry*, *170*, 609–615.

Burns, B. J., & Hoagwood, K. (Eds.). (2002). *Community treatment for youth: Evidence-based interventions for severe emotional and behavioral disorders*. New York: Oxford University Press.

Burns, B. J., Hoagwood, K., & Mrazek, P. J. (1999). Effective treatment for mental disorders in children and adolescents. *Clinical Child and Family Psychology Review*, *2*, 199–254.

De Hert, M., van Winkel, R., Wampers, M., Kane, J., van Os, J., & Peuskens, J. (2007). Remission criteria for schizophrenia: Evaluation in a large naturalistic cohort. *Schizophrenia Research*, *92*(1–3), 68–73.

Emsley, R., Chiliza, B., Asmal, L., & Lehloenya, K. (2011). The concepts of remission and recovery in schizophrenia. *Current Opinion in Psychiatry*, *24*, 114–121.

Henggeler, S. W., Rowland, M. D., Randall, J., Ward, D. M., Pickrel, S. G., Cunningham, P. B., . . . Santos, A. B. (1999). Home-based multisystemic therapy as an alternative to the hospitalization of youths in psychiatric crisis: Clinical outcomes. *Journal of the American Academy of Child and Adolescent Psychiatry*, *38*, 1331–1339.

Henggeler, S. W., Schoenwald, S. K., Rowland, M. D., & Cunningham, P. B. (2002). *Serious emotional disturbance in children and adolescents: Multisystemic therapy*. New York: Guilford Press.

Hogarty, G. E., Flesher, S., Ulrich, R., Carter, M., Greenwald, D., Poque-Geile, M., . . . Zoretich, R. (2002). Cognitive enhancement therapy for schizophrenia: Effects of a 2-year randomized trial on cognition and behavior. *Archives of General Psychiatry, 200*, 866–876.

Lambert, M., Karow, A., Leucht, S., Schimmelmann, B. G., & Naber, D. (2010). Remission in schizophrenia: Validity, frequency, predictors, and patients' perspective 5 years later. *Dialogues in Clinical Neuroscience, 12*, 393–407.

Liberman, R. P., Kopelowicz, A., Ventura, J., & Gutkind, D. (2002). Operational criteria and factors related to recovery from schizophrenia. *International Review of Psychiatry, 14*, 256–272.

Lieberman, J. A., Stroup, T. S., McEvoy, J. P., Swartz, M. S., Rosenheck, R. A., Perkins, D. O., . . . Hsaio, J. K. (2005). Effectiveness of antipsychotic drugs in patients with chronic schizophrenia. *New England Journal of Medicine, 353*, 1209–1223.

Masi, G., Mucci, M., & Pari, C. (2006). Children with schizophrenia: Clinical picture and pharmacological treatment. *CNS Drugs, 20*, 841–866.

Rowland, M. D., & Westlake, L. A. (2006). *Mental health multisystemic therapy psychiatry resource book.* Mount Pleasant, SC: MST Services.

Substance Abuse and Mental Health Services Administration. (2014). *National registry of evidence-based programs and practices.* Retrieved from http://www.nrepp.samhsa.gov/Index.aspx

Ucok, A., & Gaebel, W. (2008). Side effects of atypical antipsychotics: A brief overview. *World Psychiatry, 7*, 58–62.

CHAPTER 16

Substance Abuse Co-occurrence with Mental Health Issues

THIS CHAPTER will consider substance use and abuse, present diagnostic criteria, and discuss substance abuse co-occurrence with mental health conditions (co-occurring disorders or COD). The current status of types of drugs most used by children and adolescents will be presented and the chapter will conclude with a discussion of the evidence-based interventions for co-occurring disorders, mental illness, and substance abuse. The world of substance abuse is always changing and it is difficult for the field to keep up. What is presented in this chapter is the current state of knowledge, but social workers need to take an active role in keeping current on trends.

Adolescents use alcohol and other drugs for many reasons, including curiosity, to feel good, to reduce stress, and to feel grown up or to fit in. It is difficult to know which adolescent will experiment and stop and which will develop serious problems. Teenagers at risk for developing serious alcohol and drug problems include:

- Those with a family history of substance abuse
- Those who are depressed
- Those who have low self-esteem
- Those who feel that they don't fit in or are out of the mainstream

Substance abuse, which includes alcohol and drugs, is a health and social problem among adolescents and young adults. Substance abuse disorders are among the most common disorders in adolescents and commonly co-occur with a wide range of psychiatric disorders. Adolescents and young adults with mental health conditions have higher rates of substance-abuse-related disorders than adolescents and young adults in the general population (Anthony, Taylor, & Raffo, 2011).

Substance use disorders are associated with maladaptive use, abuse, or dependency that results in adverse social, behavioral, psychological, and physiological consequences for the child or adolescent. For youth, consequences are most frequently expressed as deterioration in peer and family relationships, decline in school attendance and academic functioning, higher levels of negative affect (depression and anxiety), and involvement in antisocial behaviors (Jordan, Scannapieco, & Vandiver, 2009).

SUBSTANCE USE IN THE GENERAL POPULATION

It is important to explore usage of alcohol and other drugs with youth, particularly those with mental health issues because substance use will exacerbate the risk of health and behavioral issues. Adolescence is a time of experimentation, and some usage of alcohol and other drugs should be expected. To get a sense of what is normal usage across the youth population, statistics will be presented across age, gender, and race.

According to the Substance Abuse and Mental Health Services Administration (SAMHSA; 2011a), more than half of Americans aged twelve or older (51.8 percent) reported being current drinkers of alcohol in the 2010 survey. Table 16.1 provides a breakdown by age, sex, and racial/ethnic group for youth who reported being current users of alcohol.

Table 16.1. Percentage of youth reporting current usage of alcohol

By age	
12–13	3.1%
16–17	24.6%
18–20	48.9%
By sex, age 12–17	
Male	13.7%
Female	13.5%
By racial/ethnic group, age 12–17	
Asian	4.8%
Black	10.8%
American Indian/Alaska Native	11.1%
Youth reporting two or more races	13.0%
Hispanic	13.9%
White	14.9%

In 2010, 10.1 percent of youth aged twelve to seventeen were current illicit drug users. Table 16.2 provides a breakdown of illicit drug use reported by these youth by substance, by sex, and by racial/ethnic group.

Given the percentages of current alcohol and drug users shown in Tables 16.1 and 16.2, it is important to understand the continuum of usage and be able to distinguish between use and abuse of alcohol and other drugs.

CONTINUUM OF ALCOHOL AND DRUG USE

Adolescents who use drugs or alcohol can be characterized along a continuum. Levels of use are generally identified as use, abuse, and dependence. For many youth and adolescents, some alcohol and drug use is normal and should be expected. Developmentally, youth are experimenting with adult-like behaviors and substance use will not generally lead to addiction. Use of drugs or alcohol by an adolescent to experiment or socialize and in moderation is usually considered substance use rather than substance abuse. For adolescents who have a mental illness and are on medication, even small amounts of alcohol or other drugs may cause physical, emotional, or social problems. So how much is too much? According to the *Diagnostic and Statistical Manual of Mental Disorders* (American Psychiatric Association, 2000, 2013) abuse and dependence are assessed by

Table 16.2. Percentage of youth aged 12–17 reporting current use of illicit drugs (SAMHSA, 2011b)

By substance	
Marijuana	7.4%
Psychotherapeutic drugs (nonmedical use)	3.0%
Inhalants (nonmedical use)	1.1%
Hallucinogens	0.9%
Cocaine	0.2%
By sex	
Male*	10.4%
Female*	9.8%
By racial/ethnic group (ages 12 or older)	
Asian	3.5%
Native Hawaiian or other Pacific Islander	5.4%
American Indian	12.5%
Alaska Native	12.1%
Black	10.7%
Hispanic	8.1%
White	9.1%

*Males were more likely than females to be current marijuana users (8.3% vs. 6.4%), whereas females were more likely than males to be current users of psychotherapeutic drugs (3.7% vs. 2.3%) and current nonmedical users of pain relievers (3.0% vs. 2.0%).

the following criteria. Abuse of alcohol or drugs includes at least one of the following factors in the last twelve months:

- Recurrent substance use resulting in failure to fulfill obligations at work, home, or school;
- Recurrent substance use in situations that are physically hazardous;
- Recurrent substance-related legal problems;
- Continued substance use despite having persistent or recurrent social or interpersonal problems caused by or exacerbated by the substance.

Dependence, also referred to as addiction, is a pattern of use that results in three or more of the following symptoms in a twelve-month period:

- Tolerance, or needing more of the drug or alcohol to get high;
- Withdrawal, in the form of physical symptoms that occur when alcohol or other drugs are not used, such as tremors, nausea, sweating, and shakiness;

- Substance taken in larger amounts and over a longer period than intended;
- Persistent desire or unsuccessful efforts to cut down or control substance use;
- A great deal of time spent in activities related to obtaining the substance, using the substance, or recovering from its effects
- Important social, occupational, or recreational activities eliminated or reduced because of substance use;
- Continued substance use despite knowledge of persistent or recurrent physical or psychological problems caused or exacerbated by the substance.

ASSESSMENT

There is significant overlap in symptoms and behaviors of adolescents who are misusing drugs or alcohol with other mental health conditions. Identification and assessment need to be accurate and comprehensive to ensure correct conclusions. The assessment involves efficient identification of substance use and related problems, psychiatric co-occurrence, and psychosocial problems. The first phase of the assessment should be the identification of a substance use disorder (SUD). Because it is often not possible or desirable to have an adolescent take a physical test such as a urinalysis or blood test to identify substance use, a brief screening instrument can be used. Once it becomes clear that the adolescent has a SUD, a more comprehensive assessment of problem severity needs to be conducted.

A screening tool is a brief self-report or interview focused on the youth's behavior, thoughts, and feelings. It usually takes five to fifteen minutes and is scored to determine if the youth is within a range that indicates the likelihood of having a substance abuse problem. There are many screening instruments available. Some examples of standardized self-report screening tools are presented below. Comprehensive assessment will be discussed in the following section.

Brief Screening Instruments

A specialized six-item screen in the public domain, CRAFFT (Car, Relax, Alone, Forget, Friends, Trouble) is designed to be administered verbally during a routine interview to address both alcohol and drug use. (For more information, see http://www.projectcork.org/clinical_tools/pdf/CRAFFT.pdf). Following are some sample questions:

- Have you ever ridden in a car driven by someone (including yourself) who was high or using alcohol or drugs?
- Do you ever forget things you did while using alcohol or drugs?
- Do your family or friends ever tell you that you should cut down on your drinking or drug use?

The Rutgers Alcohol Problem Index (http://adai.washington.edu/instruments/pdf/Rutgers_Alcohol_Problem_Index_210.pdf) is an eighteen-item screen tool that assesses adolescent problem drinking and related negative consequences (White & Labouvie, 1989). Each of the sample items listed below is used to assess the frequency of the behavior in relationship to alcohol use during the past three years:

- Had withdrawal symptoms, that is, felt sick because you stopped or cut down on drinking?
- Suddenly found yourself in a place that you could not remember getting to?
- Felt that you needed more alcohol than you used to in order to get the same effect?

The Michigan Alcohol Screening Test (https://outcometracker.org/library/MAST.pdf) contains twenty-five items that provide a general measure of problem severity. Three sample questions are provided below:

- Do you feel you are a normal drinker? ("normal"—drinking as much or less than most other people)
- Have you ever awakened the morning after drinking the night before and found that you could not remember a part of the evening?
- Does any near relative or close friend ever worry or complain about your drinking?

Comprehensive Assessment

The outcome of the brief screening determines the need for a more comprehensive assessment. The comprehensive assessment explores the extent and nature of the substance involvement, psychosocial issues, and co-occurring mental health disorders. It is important to consider developmental domains such as cognitive, emotional, physical, and social. This assessment provides the more extensive information needed to determine the most appropriate intervention. Included in the determination of the intervention are treatment setting (e.g., inpatient or outpatient); type of intervention (e.g., family therapy, medications, or group therapy); and intensity, frequency, and type of contacts with therapist or resources. Specialized training is required to administer comprehensive as well as brief screening tools. The following are some examples of comprehensive assessments:

- The Global Appraisal of Individual Needs (GAIN) is a semi-structured interview that measures recent and lifetime functioning in several areas, including substance use, legal and school functioning, and psychiatric symptoms. The comprehensiveness and multidimensionality of the GAIN require a relatively long administration time and a lengthy and detailed training. (For more information, see http://www.gaincc.org.)

- The Teen Addiction Severity Index (T-ASI) is a semi-structured interview that consists of seven content areas: chemical use, school status, employment-support status, family relationships, legal status, peer-social relationships, and psychiatric status. Adolescent and interviewer severity ratings are elicited on a five-point scale for each content area. (More information is available from http://pubs.niaaa.nih.gov /publications/AssessingAlcohol/InstrumentPDFs/70_T-ASI.pdf.)

- The Personal Experience Inventory (PEI) is a self-administered, multi-scale questionnaire. It consists of several scales that measure drug use problem severity, psychosocial risk, and response distortion tendencies. Supplemental problem screens measure eating disorders, suicide potential, physical/sexual abuse, and parental history of drug abuse. (More information is available at http://www.wpspublish.com/store/p/ 2905/personal-experience-inventory-pei.)

INDICATORS OF SUBSTANCE ABUSE AND MENTAL HEALTH DISORDERS

Often an adolescent's behavior or appearance can provide signs of a substance abuse or mental health disorder. Adolescents experiencing depression, bulimia, or early stages of substance use may be actively trying to conceal their activity from adults. Research has shown that these problems are often difficult for caregivers and other adults to identify (Levitt, Saka, Romanelli, & Hoagwood, 2007; Logan & King, 2002). The National Institute of Mental Health and SAMHSA developed a toolkit (http://store.samhsa.gov/shin/content/SMA12-4700/SMA12 -4700.pdf) to help human service organizations identify signs that indicate the need to take action and address mental health or substance use conditions in children and adolescents. The following action signs are identified:

- Feeling very sad or withdrawn for more than two weeks;
- Seriously trying to harm or kill oneself, or making plans to do so;
- Sudden overwhelming fear for no reason, sometimes with a racing heart or fast breathing;
- Involvement in many fights, using a weapon, or wanting to badly hurt others;
- Severe out-of-control behavior that can hurt oneself or others;
- Not eating, throwing up, or using laxatives to lose weight;
- Intense worries or fears that get in the way of daily activities;
- Extreme difficulty concentrating or staying still that puts one in physical danger or causes school failure;
- Repeated use of drugs or alcohol;
- Severe mood swings that cause problems in relationships;
- Drastic changes in behavior or personality.

As reported by Jordan et al. (2009), indicators of substance-induced disorders for adolescents include but are not limited to physical signs (e.g., fatigue, repeated health complaints, red and glazed eyes, and lasting cough), emotional signs (e.g., personality change, irritability, irresponsible behavior, sudden mood changes, low self-esteem, poor judgment, and depression), family issues (e.g., starting arguments, breaking rules, and withdrawing from family activities), school problems (e.g., drop in grades, change in attitude about school, many absences, truancy, and discipline problems), and social problems (e.g., engaging in criminal activities, theft, or vandalism; changes in dress style or appearance; and new friends who share similar signs).

Signs of substance use must be considered in the context of the adolescent's development and situation. Many indicators are normal adolescent behaviors, but if the youth is exhibiting several over a period of time, it is important to assess substance use. Some other general signs of alcohol or drug use are listed in Table 16.3.

COMMONLY USED DRUGS AND ALCOHOL

In addition to understanding the signs and symptoms of substance use, you should know the different types of drugs, how to identify them, and their health effects. Also important is knowing the street or slang terms and how they are administered so you can communicate with the adolescent. As shown in Table 16.4, substances can generally be categorized into seven areas: alcohol, cannabinoids, stimulants, opiates, club drugs, dissociative drugs, and other. Adolescents are also increasingly abusing prescription drugs. Prescription drugs will be discussed in the following subsection.

Table 16.3. General signs of alcohol or drug use

Home
• Loss of interest in family activities
• Disrespect for family rules
• Verbal or physical abuse
• Disappearance of valuable items or money
• Not telling where they are going
• Constant excuses for behavior

School
• Sudden drop in grades
• Truancy or always being late to school
• Loss of interest in learning
• Poor work performance
• Defiance of authority
• Reduced memory and attention span
• Poor attitude toward sports or other extracurricular activities

Physical and emotional signs
• Different friends
• Smell of alcohol or marijuana on breath or body
• Unexplainable mood swings and behavior
• Overreaction to criticism or rebelliousness
• Negativity, argumentativeness, paranoia or confusion, destructiveness, or anxiety
• Feeling overly tired or being hyperactive
• Drastic weight gain or loss
• Cheating or stealing

Table 16.4. Characteristics of commonly abused alcohol and drugs

Category	Street name	Administered	Acute effects	Health risk
Alcohol				
Liquor, beer, and wine		Swallowed	Euphoria, mild stimulation, relaxation, lowered inhibitions, slurred speech, nausea, loss of coordination	Increased risk of injuries, violence, fetal damage, depression, hypertension, liver and heart disease, addiction
Cannabinoids				
Marijuana	Blunt, dope, ganja, grass, herb, joint, bud, Mary Jane, pot, reefer, green, weed	Smoked, swallowed	Euphoria, relaxation, slowed reaction time, distorted sensory perception, impaired balance and coordination, increased heart rate and appetite, anxiety, panic attacks, psychosis	Cough, frequent respiratory infections, possible mental health decline, addiction
Hashish	Boom, gangster, hash, hash oil, hemp	Smoked or swallowed	Euphoria, relaxation, slowed reaction time, distorted sensory perception, impaired balance and coordination, increased heart rate and appetite, anxiety, panic attacks, psychosis	Cough, frequent respiratory infections, possible mental health decline, addiction
Opioids				
Heroin	Smack, horse, brown sugar, dope, H, junk, skag, skunk, white horse, China white, cheese (with over the counter cold medicine and antihistamine)	Injected, smoked, snorted	Euphoria, drowsiness, impaired coordination, dizziness, confusion, nausea, sedation, feeling of heaviness in the body, slowed or arrested breathing	Constipation, endocarditis, hepatitis, HIV, addiction, fatal overdose
Opium	Big O, black stuff, block, gum, hop	Swallowed, smoked	Euphoria, drowsiness, impaired coordination, dizziness, confusion, nausea, sedation, feeling of heaviness in the body, slowed or arrested breathing	Constipation, endocarditis, hepatitis, HIV, addiction, fatal overdose

Table 16.4. (Continued)

Category	Street name	Administered	Acute effects	Health risk
Stimulants				
Cocaine	Blow, bump, C, candy, Charlie, coke, crack, flake, rock, snow, toot	Snorted, smoked, injected	Increased heart rate, blood pressure, body temperature, and metabolism; feelings of exhilaration; increased energy and mental alertness; tremors; reduced appetite; irritability; anxiety; panic; paranoia; violent behavior; psychosis	Nasal damage from snorting, weight loss, insomnia, cardiac or cardiovascular complications, stroke, seizures, addiction
Amphetamines	Bennies, black beauties, crosses, hearts, LA turnaround, speed, truck drivers, uppers	Swallowed, snorted, smoked, injected	Increased heart rate, blood pressure, body temperature, and metabolism; feelings of exhilaration; increased energy and mental alertness; tremors; reduced appetite; irritability; anxiety; panic; paranoia; violent behavior; psychosis	Weight loss, insomnia, cardiac or cardiovascular complications, stroke, seizures, addiction
Methamphetamines	Meth, ice, crank, chalk, crystal, fire, glass, go fast, speed	Swallowed, snorted, smoked, injected	Increased heart rate, blood pressure, body temperature, and metabolism; feelings of exhilaration; increased energy and mental alertness; tremors; reduced appetite; irritability; anxiety; panic; paranoia; violent behavior; psychosis	Severe dental problems, weight loss, insomnia, cardiac or cardiovascular complications, stroke, seizures, addiction
Club Drugs				
MDMA (methylenedioxy-methamphetamine)	Ecstasy, Adam, clarity, Eve, lover's speed, peace, uppers	Swallowed, snorted, injected	Mild hallucinogenic effects, increased tactile sensitivity, empathic feelings, lowered inhibition, anxiety, chills, sweating, teeth clenching, muscle cramping	Sleep disturbances, depression, impaired memory, hyperthermia, addiction

Table 16.4. (Continued)

Category	Street name	Administered	Acute effects	Health risk
Flunitrazepam (associated with sexual assault)	Rohypnol, forget-me pill, Mexican Valium, R2, roach, Roche, roofies, roofinol, rape, rophies	Swallowed, snorted	Mild hallucinogenic effects, increased tactile sensitivity, empathic feelings, lowered inhibition, anxiety, chills, sweating, teeth clenching, muscle cramping, sedation, muscle relaxation, confusion, memory loss, dizziness, impaired coordination	Addiction
GHB (gamma-hydroxybutyric acid; associated with sexual assault)	G, Georgia home boy, grievous bodily harm, liquid ecstasy, soap, scoop, goop, liquid x	Swallowed	Mild hallucinogenic effects, increased tactile sensitivity, empathic feelings, lowered inhibition, anxiety, chills, sweating, teeth clenching, muscle cramping	Unconsciousness, seizures, coma
Dissociative drugs				
Ketamine	Ketalar SV, cat valium, K, Special K, vitamin K	Injected, snorted, smoked	Feelings of being separate from one's body and environment, impaired motor function, impaired memory, delirium, respiratory depression and arrest, death	Anxiety, tremors, numbness, memory loss, nausea
PCP and analogs	Phencyclidine, angel dust, boat, hog, love boat, peace pill	Swallowed, smoked, injected	Psychosis, aggression, violence, slurred speech, loss of coordination, hallucinations, feelings of being separate from one's body and environment, impaired motor function, impaired memory, delirium, respiratory depression and arrest, death	Anxiety, tremors, numbness, memory loss, nausea

Prescription Drug Use among Adolescents

Many adolescents are under the misconception that prescription drugs are safer than street or illicit drugs. The use of psychotherapeutic drugs makes up a larger part of the overall U.S. drug problem than was true in the 1990s. After alcohol and marijuana, prescription and over the counter drugs are among the most commonly abused drugs by twelfth graders (National Institute on Drug Abuse, n.d.), partly because there is an increase in prescription drugs overall and partly because use of illicit drugs is down. Young people seem less concerned about using prescription drugs because of their legitimate widespread use. Additionally, adolescents and young adults are aware of only the positive benefits and not the dangers of using prescription drugs for nonmedical reasons.

Prescription drug abuse occurs when someone takes a medication prescribed for someone else or takes his or her own prescription in a dosage other than what was prescribed. Young people often abuse prescription drugs belonging to friends or relatives to get high, to treat pain, or to help them study or stay alert longer. Often teens will use the drug in a different form or dosage to get high quicker. Most prescription drugs come in pill form. Young adults who abuse prescription drugs will crush the pill and then swallow, sniff, or inject it, which may cause serious side effects or addiction. For example, when oxycodone (OxyContin) is crushed and inhaled, a twelve-hour dose hits the central nervous system all at once, which increases the risk of addiction and overdose (National Institute on Drug Abuse, 2014).

Commonly Abused Prescription Drugs

Similar to illicit drugs, prescription drugs that are abused fall into categories. Table 16.5 will break them into the following categories: depressants, opioids and morphine derivatives, stimulants and other compounds.

TREATMENT OF CO-OCCURRING DISORDERS

Treatment of mental illness along with a substance abuse disorder is a relatively new field, and evidence-based practices developed specifically for clients with co-occurring disorders are limited. Therefore it is important to consider evidence-based practices developed solely for either mental health or substance abuse. The current state of the science highlights the need for evidence-based

Table 16.5.   Characteristics of commonly abused prescription drugs

Category	Commercial and street names	Administered	Acute effects	Health risk
Depressants				
Barbiturates	Amytal, Nembutal, Seconal, Phenobarbital; barbs, reds, red birds, tooies, yellows	Injected, swallowed	Euphoria, unusual excitement, fever, sedation, reduced anxiety, feelings of well-being, lowered inhibitions, slurred speech, poor concentration, confusion, dizziness, impaired coordination and memory	Lowered blood pressure, slowed breathing, tolerance, withdrawal, addiction, increased risk of respiratory distress and death when combined with alcohol
Benzodiazepines	Ativan, Halcion, Librium, Valium, Xanax; candy, downers, sleeping pills, tranks	Swallowed	Sedation, reduced anxiety, feelings of well-being, lowered inhibitions, slurred speech, poor concentration, confusion, dizziness, impaired coordination and memory	Addiction, worsening of some breathing problems, possible birth defects for pregnant women, in the elderly may lead to falling
Sleep medication	Ambien, Sonata, Lunesta; forget-me pill, Mexican Valium, R2, Roche, roofies, roofinaol, rope, rophies	Swallowed, snorted	Sedation, reduced anxiety, feelings of well-being, lowered inhibitions, slurred speech, poor concentration, confusion, dizziness, impaired coordination and memory	Burning or tingling in the hands, arms, feet, or legs; changes in appetite, difficulty keeping balance, dizziness, daytime drowsiness, mental slowing or problems with attention or memory
Opioids/morphine				
Codeine	Empirin with Codeine, Fiorinal with Codeine, Robitussin A-C, Tylenol with Codeine; Captain Cody, schoolboy	Injected, swallowed	Pain relief, euphoria, drowsiness, sedation, weakness, dizziness, nausea, impaired coordination, confusion, dry mouth, itching, sweating, clammy skin, constipation	Slowed or arrested breathing, lowered pulse and blood pressure, tolerance, addiction, unconsciousness, coma, death (risk of death increased when combined with alcohol or other central nervous system depressants)
Morphine	Roxanol, Duramorph; Miss Emma, monkey, white stuff	Injected, swallowed, smoked	Pain relief, euphoria, drowsiness, sedation, weakness, dizziness, nausea, impaired coordination, confusion, dry mouth, itching, sweating, clammy skin, constipation	Slowed or arrested breathing, lowered pulse and blood pressure, tolerance, addiction, unconsciousness, coma, death (risk of death increased when combined with alcohol or other central nervous system depressants)

Table 16.5.   (Continued)

Category	Commercial and street names	Administered	Acute effects	Health risk
Methadone	Methadose, Dolophine; fizzies, amidone	Swallowed, injected	Significant overdose risk when used improperly, pain relief, euphoria, drowsiness, sedation, weakness, dizziness, nausea, impaired coordination, confusion, dry mouth, itching, sweating, clammy skin, constipation	Slowed or arrested breathing, lowered pulse and blood pressure, tolerance, addiction, unconsciousness, coma, death (risk of death increased when combined with alcohol or other central nervous system depressants)
Fentanyl and analogs	Actiq, Duragesic, Sublimaze; Apache, China girl, China white, dance fever, friend, goodfella, jackpot, murder 8, TNT, Tango and Cash	Injected, smoked, snorted	80 to 100 times more potent analgesic than morphine; pain relief, euphoria, drowsiness, sedation, weakness, dizziness, nausea, impaired coordination, confusion, dry mouth, itching, sweating, clammy skin, constipation	Slowed or arrested breathing, lowered pulse and blood pressure, tolerance, addiction, unconsciousness, coma, death (risk of death increased when combined with alcohol or other central nervous system depressants)
Other opioid pain relievers				
Oxycodone HCL, Hydrocodone Bitartrate, Hydromorphone, Oxymorphone, Meperidine, Propoxyphene	Tylox, Oxycontin, Percodan, Percocet, Vicodin, Lortab, Demerol; Oxy, O.C., oxycotton, kicker, hillbilly, percs, smack, smurfs, footballs, stop signs, blue heaven, blues, Mrs. O	Chewed, swallowed, snorted, injected, suppositories	Muscle relaxation, high abuse potential, pain relief, euphoria, drowsiness, sedation, weakness, dizziness, nausea, impaired coordination, confusion, dry mouth, itching, sweating, clammy skin, constipation	Slowed or arrested breathing, lowered pulse and blood pressure, tolerance, addiction, unconsciousness, coma, death (risk of death increased when combined with alcohol or other central nervous system depressants)
Stimulants				
Amphetamines	Biphetamine, Dexedrine, Adderall; bennies, black beauties, crosses, hearts, LA turnaround, speed, truck drivers, uppers	Injected, swallowed, smoked, snorted	Feelings of exhilaration, increased energy, mental alertness	Increased heart rate, blood pressure, and metabolism; reduced appetite; weight loss; nervousness; insomnia; seizures; heart attack; stroke; rapid breathing; tremor; loss of coordination; irritability; panic; hallucinations; impulsive behavior; addiction

Table 16.5. (Continued)

Category	Commercial and street names	Administered	Acute effects	Health risk
Methylphenidate	Concerta, Ritalin; JIF, MPH, R-ball, Skippy, the smart drug, Vitamin R	Injected, swallowed, snorted	Feelings of exhilaration, increased energy, mental alertness	Increased or decreased blood pressure, increased heart rate and metabolism, reduced appetite, weight loss, digestive problems, nervousness, insomnia, seizures, heart attack, stroke
Other compounds				
Dextromethorphan (DXM)	Found in some cough and cold medicines; Robotripping, Robo, Triple C	Swallowed	Euphoria, slurred speech	Increased heart rate and blood pressure, dizziness, nausea, vomiting, confusion, paranoia, distorted visual perceptions, impaired motor function

thinking in making both programmatic and clinical decisions in the treatment of people with co-occurring disorders (SAMHSA, 2014).

At the *treatment level*, interventions that have their own evidence to support them as evidence-based practices are frequently a part of a comprehensive and integrated response to persons with co-occurring disorders. These interventions, which have been described previously in this book, include the following:

- Psychopharmacological interventions (e.g., desipramine and bupropion for people with cocaine use disorders and depression [Kranzler & Ciraulo, 2005])
- Motivational interventions (e.g., motivational enhancement therapy [Miller & Rollnick, 2013])
- Cognitive-behavioral interventions (e.g., contingency management [Higgins, Silverman, & Heil, 2007; Roth, Brunette, & Green, 2005])

At the *program level*, three models have an evidence base for producing positive clinical outcomes for persons with co-occurring existing disorders: the modified therapeutic community, integrated dual disorders treatment, and assertive community treatment. The modified therapeutic community (MTC; De Leon, 1993; De Leon, Sacks, Staines, & McKendrick, 2000; Sacks, Banks, McKendrick, & Sacks, 2008) for persons with co-occurring disorders is a twelve- to eighteen-month residential treatment program. Developed for individuals with co-occurring substance use disorders and mental disorders, the MTC is a structured and active program based on community-as-method (that is, the community is the treatment agent) and mutual peer self-help. It is a comprehensive treatment model that adapts the traditional therapeutic community in response to the psychiatric symptoms, cognitive impairments, and reduced level of functioning of the client with co-occurring disorders. Treatment encompasses four stages (admission, primary treatment, live-in reentry, and live-out reentry) that correspond to stages within the recovery process. The staged format allows gradual progress, rewarding improvement with increased independence and responsibility. Goals, objectives, and expected outcomes are established for each stage and are integrated in an individual treatment plan with goals specific to each client. Staff members function as role models, rational authorities, and guides (Center for Substance Abuse Treatment, 2007).

Research has strongly indicated that, to recover fully, a person with a co-occurring disorder needs treatment for both problems. Integrated dual disorder treatments provide assistance for each condition, helping people recover from both in one setting and at the same time.

Key to integrated dual disorder treatment is the inclusion of assistance beyond standard therapy or medication, such as assertive outreach, job and housing assistance, family counseling, and even money and relationship management. This personalized treatment is viewed as long term and can be begun at any stage of recovery. A strengths-based approach is at the foundation of integrated treatment (SAMHSA, 2014).

Assertive community treatment is designed as a service delivery model in which a team of professionals assumes responsibility for providing the specific mix of services that each person needs at the appropriate frequency and intensity and for the appropriate length of time. Team members are available twenty-four hours a day, seven days a week. Services are provided in the community in places and situations where problems arise, rather than in an office or clinic setting. Interventions are integrated through collaboration among team members.

REFERENCES

American Psychiatric Association. (2000). *Diagnostic and statistical manual of mental disorders* (4th ed., text rev.). Washington, DC: Author.

American Psychiatric Association. (2013). *Diagnostic and statistical manual of mental disorders* (5th ed.). Washington, DC: Author.

Anthony, E. K., Taylor, S. A., & Raffo, Z. (2011). Early intervention for substance abuse among youth and young adults with mental health conditions: An exploration of community mental health practices. *Administration and Policy in Mental Health and Mental Health Services Research, 38*, 131–141. doi:10.1007/s10488–010–0308-x

Center for Substance Abuse Treatment. (2007). *Understanding evidence-based practices for co-occurring disorders* (COCE Overview Paper 5, DHHS Publication No. SMA 07–4278). Rockville, MD: Substance Abuse and Mental Health Services Administration.

De Leon, G. (1993). Modified therapeutic communities for co-occurring substance abuse and psychiatric disorders. In J. Solomon, S. Zimberg, & E. Shollar (Eds.), *Dual diagnosis: Evaluation, treatment, training, and program development* (pp. 137–156). New York: Plenum.

De Leon, G., Sacks, S., Staines, G., & McKendrick, K. (2000). Modified therapeutic community for homeless mentally ill chemical abusers: Treatment outcomes. *American Journal of Drug and Alcohol Abuse, 26*, 461–480.

Higgins, S. T., Silverman, K., & Heil, S. H. (Eds.). (2007). *Contingency management in substance abuse treatment.* New York: Guilford Press.

Jordan, C., Scannapieco, M., & Vandiver, V. L. (2009). Health promotion strategies for the mental health needs of children and families. In V. L. Vandiver (Ed.), *Integrating health promotion and mental health: An introduction to policies, principles, and practices.* New York: Oxford University Press.

Kranzler, H. R., & Ciraulo, D. A. (Eds.). (2005). *Clinical manual of addiction psychopharmacology.* Arlington, VA: American Psychiatric Publishing.

Levitt, J. M., Saka, N., Romanelli, L. H., & Hoagwood, K. (2007). Early identification of mental health problems in schools: The status of instrumentation. *Journal of School Psychology, 45*, 163–191.

Logan, D. E., & King, C. A. (2002). Parental identification of depression and mental health service use among depressed adolescents. *Journal of the American Academy of Child and Adolescent Psychiatry, 41*, 296–304.

Miller, W. R., & Rollnick, S. (2013). *Motivational interviewing: Helping people change.* (3rd ed.). New York: Guilford Press.

National Institute on Drug Abuse. (n.d.). *Topics in brief: Prescription drug abuse.* Retrieved from http://www.drugabuse.gov/publications/term/163/TopicsInBrief

National Institute on Drug Abuse. (2014). *NIDA for teens.* Retrieved from http://teens.drugabuse.gov/facts/facts_mj1.php

Roth, R. M., Brunette, M. F., & Green, A. I. (2005). Treatment of substance use disorder in schizophrenia: A unifying neurobiological mechanism? *Current Psychiatry Reports, 7,* 283–291.

Sacks, S., Banks, S., McKendrick, K., & Sacks, J. Y. (2008). Modified therapeutic community for co-occurring disorders: A summary of four studies. *Journal of Substance Abuse Treatment, 34,* 112–122.

Substance Abuse and Mental Health Services Administration. (2011a). *Identifying mental health and substance use problems of children and adolescents: A guide for child-serving organizations* (HHS Publication No. SMA 12–4670). Rockville, MD: Author.

Substance Abuse and Mental Health Services Administration. (2011b). *Results from the 2010 National Survey on Drug Use and Health: Summary of national findings* (NSDUH Series H-41, HHS Publication No. SMA 11–4658). Rockville, MD: Author.

Substance Abuse and Mental Health Services Administration. (2014). *National registry of evidence-based programs and practices.* Available from http://www.nrepp.samhsa.gov/Index.aspx

White, H. R., & Labouvie, E. W. (1989). Towards the assessment of adolescent problem drinking. *Journal of Studies on Alcohol, 50,* 30–37.

CHAPTER 17

Children and Adolescents with Mental Illness and the Education System

SCHOOL IS AN IMPORTANT ASPECT of all youths' and children's lives. They spend most of each school day in the classroom. It is often not until the child enters the school system that mental health issues are discovered. School-teachers, social workers, nurses, and other personnel are in an exceptional position to identify child mental health issues because they are in sustained contact and often have a trusting relationship with children. Schools also provide a safe and expected place to address behaviors resulting from mental health issues. At the end of the chapter we will share several evidence-informed interventions designed for use in schools, supporting the importance of the school setting for the child or adolescent who is struggling.

School can be a challenging place for children experiencing emotional or behavioral problems. If a child is not in the most appropriate setting

and receiving the most appropriate supports, there can be serious, lifelong consequences. The caregivers of these children can also find the school system challenging, particularly if they do not understand their child's rights and how to
advocate for their child's needs. What are the educational system's obligations
for dealing with children who have a mental health problem?

There are two federal laws that protect children with disabilities. The first
is the Individuals with Disabilities Education Act (IDEA; 2004). This act sets
achievement standards and provides guidance to schools on how to help students
achieve these standards. The Individuals with Disabilities Education Act requires
the educational system to ensure that eligible children with disabilities, including
mental health disabilities, receive the same educational opportunities as children
without disabilities.

The second federal provision is included in Section 504 of the Rehabilitation
Act of 1973 (1973). This is a federal civil rights law that prohibits discrimination
against people with disabilities. Under this law, children with disabilities are
afforded the right to the same educational programs and experiences as nondis-
abled children. In order to ensure this, schools must make necessary accommodations to allow children with disabilities the same opportunities as other children.
All children with a disability are covered by Section 504. To be covered under
IDEA, a child must meet certain eligibility criteria.

INDIVIDUALS WITH DISABILITIES EDUCATION ACT

The Individuals with Disabilities Education Act requires that special education
and related services be made available free of charge to every eligible child with
a disability, including preschoolers (ages 3–21). These services are specially
designed to address the child's individual needs associated with the disability—
in this case, emotional disturbance, as defined by IDEA (and further specified by
states). In recent school years, more than 490,000 children and youth received
these services to address their individual needs related to emotional disturbance.

Each year, over six million children from three to twenty-one years old
receive special education and related services. Of those, nearly 1 in 12 children
receive the services because of an emotional disturbance. The Individuals with
Disabilities Education Act spells out the requirement for schools to provide services to children when their disability interferes with their ability to learn. State
educational laws define how children should be identified and served under

IDEA. The federal government provides state funds to help pay for accommodations that are needed to help a child with special needs receive an appropriate education in the least restrictive situation. If states do not comply with IDEA, they stand to lose those federal funds.

The first step for a child to receive special education services under IDEA is a complete evaluation by qualified school professionals to determine if the child has a mental health problem covered under the state's educational plan and if that problem is interfering with the child's ability to learn in a regular classroom setting. This evaluation is provided free of charge in public schools.

Once the evaluation is completed, the caregiver(s) and school personnel meet to review the results and determine whether special educational supports and services are needed, and if so, what types of supports and services are appropriate. If the family disagrees with the findings of the evaluation or the recommendations, it can request an independent evaluation by qualified professionals that do not work for the school.

Definition of a Child with a Disability under IDEA

There are various disability categories under which a child may be found eligible for special education and related services:

- Autism
- Deafness
- Deaf-blindness
- Developmental delay
- Emotional disturbance
- Hearing impairment
- Intellectual disability
- Multiple disabilities
- Orthopedic impairment
- Other health impairment
- Specific learning disability
- Speech or language impairment
- Traumatic brain injury
- Visual impairment including blindness

If a student is deemed eligible, and the family agrees to special education accommodations, school personnel including teachers and counselors have a face-to-face meeting with the family and any other persons the family would like to participate. It can be helpful for the family to have a family advocate who understands IDEA to attend the meeting with them. Together, the team should develop an individualized educational program (IEP) that spells out educational goals, short-term objectives, and services or accommodations to be provided through the school. Accommodations may include alterations in assignments, changes in expectations for the child to receive a passing grade, modification to the environment to reduce distractions or temptations, or an individualized behavior plan.

A meeting should be held with the team at least once a year to review the goals, objectives, and services; determine if they are meeting the needs of the child; and set new goals and objectives. Meetings can be requested earlier if the plan needs to be changed to better meet the child's educational needs. In addition to an annual IEP meeting, the child should be reevaluated at least once every three years and no more than once a year to determine continued eligibility and to address any new needs. If a family does not feel that the child's needs are being met, or if the child's rights are being violated, the family can request due process.

EMOTIONAL AND BEHAVIORAL PROBLEMS

When children with emotional or behavioral problems exhibit behaviors that interfere with their ability to learn, or with the ability of other children around them to learn, a behavioral intervention plan should be put in place. An assessment should be conducted to determine the type of behavior and its frequency and duration, as well as the situations under which it does or does not occur. The behavioral plan is then developed to prevent the problem behavior from occurring. A common strategy is to use a token system that allows the child to earn tokens when the problem behavior does not occur and to lose tokens when it does. The child can accrue tokens that can be used to purchase a privilege or reward. The reward must be something that is important to the specific child and must be delivered in increments based on the child's age and maturity level. For instance, a first grader should not have to wait a month before earning a reward.

INTERVENTION STRATEGIES

Schools afford professionals who work in the school system a unique opportunity to intervene with children who have experienced mental health issues. Prior to entering school, children may have experienced abuse for years. Parents may not have had any prior assistance with learning new and effective ways of child rearing or support in overcoming the many challenges of raising children with limited resources. The school can begin to provide the needed positive and secure relationships with peers and adults and social support and connection to other forms of social support for the family. Teachers can provide opportunities for personal development, fostering accomplishment, and boosting the child's self-esteem and feelings of mastery. They can help children build self-confidence and navigate the process of developing peer relationships.

All schools have children at risk of mental health issues or children with a mental health issue. These children often have difficulty learning and consequently it is difficult for the classroom teacher to manage their behaviors. Additionally, many children, particularly in large urban areas, are in foster or kinship care and require special attention from school personnel, Child Protective Services, and other mental health workers. In a time of drastic budget cuts to both educational and mental health systems, building alliances to address intervention needs of children identified as having mental health issues is critical to the mission of the school system, the education of children, and the mission of mental health agencies, as well as the safety and well-being of the child. The school social worker and other mental health professionals must be at the forefront of coordinating alliances and working with other social service agencies in addressing the needs of school-aged children.

School-based interventions can take many forms. Partnering with mental health agencies to establish programs will help to ensure that children at risk are properly identified. Often local mental health agencies are in a better position to be aware of community resources.

Children who receive intervention services through school-based alliances have been found to improve their school performance and their attendance and to have fewer behavior problems (U.S. Department of Health and Human Services, 2008). Social workers interested in building school-based alliances may want to refer to the elements of building an effective alliance using an approach based on the identified problem the alliance has chosen:

1. *Direct services to at-risk children and families.* These may include interventions such as home visits, individual or group counseling, mentoring, support groups, social events, and tutoring. Examples include:

   a. After-school programs focusing on social, recreational, educational or therapeutic issues;

   b. Problem-solving, assertiveness training, or conflict resolution programs;

   c. Mentoring programs using adults for educational and social development;

   d. Services for special needs children that focus on developmental and educational screening and advocacy for services such as transportation.

2. *Development of resource guides for school personnel.* Mental health agencies often have directories of community services relevant to the needs of at-risk children in the school setting. Through the collaboration, a resource guide specific to the needs of school personnel can be developed that addresses appropriate referral sources for families and children at risk of maltreatment.

EVIDENCE-INFORMED INTERVENTIONS

There are many evidence-informed school-based interventions directed at improving children's and adolescents' mental health. The following interventions selected from the National Registry of Evidence-based Programs and Practices (Substance Abuse and Mental Health Services Administration, 2014) are associated with middle childhood and adolescence:

- *All Stars* is a school-based program for middle school students (eleven to fourteen years old) that is designed to prevent and delay the onset of high-risk behaviors such as drug use, violence, and premature sexual activity.

- *American Indian Life Skills Development/Zuni Life Skills Development.* Suicide is the second leading cause of death among American Indians from fifteen to twenty-four years old, according to Centers for Disease Control and Prevention (2014). The estimated rate of completed suicides among American Indians in this age group is about three times higher than that among comparably aged U.S. youth overall (37.4 vs. 11.4 per 100,000, respectively).

- The *Anti-Defamation League (ADL) Peer Training Program* is an antibias and diversity training program intended for use in middle and high schools. The program prepares select students to be peer trainers.

- *Building Assets—Reducing Risks* (BARR) is a multifaceted school-based prevention program designed to decrease the incidence of substance abuse (tobacco, alcohol, and other drugs), academic failure, truancy, and disciplinary incidents among ninth grade youth.

- *CARE* (Care, Assess, Respond, Empower), formerly called Counselors CARE (C-CARE) and Measure of Adolescent Potential for Suicide (MAPS), is a high-school-based suicide prevention program targeting high-risk youth.

- *CAST* (Coping and Support Training) is a high-school-based suicide prevention program targeting youth from fourteen to nineteen years old that delivers life skills training and social support in a small group format (six to eight students per group).

- The *Challenging Horizons Program* (CHP) is a school-based set of interventions for middle/junior high school students with attention deficit hyperactivity disorder. Building on behavioral and cognitive theories about the nature of the disorder, CHP aims to provide a safe learning environment enhanced by supportive counseling relationships between students and staff.

- The *Children of Divorce Intervention Program* (CODIP) is a school-based preventive intervention delivered to groups of children from ages five to fourteen who are dealing with the challenges of parental separation and divorce.

- The *Cognitive Behavioral Intervention for Trauma in Schools* (CBITS) program is a school-based group and individual intervention designed to reduce symptoms of posttraumatic stress disorder, depression, and behavioral problems; improve peer and parent support; and enhance coping skills among students exposed to traumatic life events, such as community and school violence, physical abuse, domestic violence, accidents, and natural disasters.

- The Columbia University *TeenScreen Program* identifies middle school and high school youth in need of mental health services due to risk for suicide and undetected mental illness. The program's main objective is to assist in the early identification of problems that might not otherwise come to the attention of professionals.

- *Fourth R: Skills for Youth Relationships* is a curriculum for eighth and ninth grade students that is designed to promote healthy and safe behaviors related to dating, bullying, sexuality, and substance use.
- *Interpersonal Psychotherapy for Depressed Adolescents* (IPT-A) is a short-term, manual-driven outpatient treatment intervention that focuses on the current interpersonal problems of adolescents (aged twelve to eighteen years) with mild to moderate depression.
- *Keepin' It REAL* is a multicultural, school-based substance use prevention program for students from twelve to fourteen years old. It uses a ten-lesson curriculum taught by trained classroom teachers in forty-five-minute sessions over ten weeks, with booster sessions delivered in the following school year.
- *The Leadership Program's Violence Prevention Project* (VPP) is a school-based intervention for early and middle adolescents. It is designed to prevent conflict and violence by improving conflict resolution skills, altering norms about using aggression and violence (including lowering tolerance for violence), and improving behavior in the school and community.
- *LEADS* (Linking Education and Awareness of Depression and Suicide): *For Youth* is a curriculum for high school students in ninth through twelfth grades that is designed to increase knowledge of depression and suicide, modify perceptions of depression and suicide, increase knowledge of suicide prevention resources, and improve intentions to engage in help-seeking behaviors.
- *LifeSkills Training* (LST) is a school-based program that aims to prevent alcohol, tobacco, and marijuana use and violence by targeting the major social and psychological factors that promote the initiation of substance use and other risky behaviors.
- The *Michigan Model for Health* is a comprehensive and sequential health education curriculum that aims to give students aged five to nineteen years (grades K–12) the knowledge and skills needed to practice and maintain healthy behaviors and lifestyles.
- The *Model Adolescent Suicide Prevention Program* (MASPP) is a public-health-oriented suicidal behavior prevention and intervention

program originally developed for a small American Indian tribe in rural New Mexico to target high rates of suicide among its adolescents and young adults.

- *Nurturing Parenting Programs* (NPP) are family-based programs for the prevention and treatment of child abuse and neglect. The programs were developed to help families who have been identified by child welfare agencies for past child abuse and neglect or who are at high risk for child abuse and neglect.

- *Peaceful Alternatives to Tough Situations* (PATTS) is a school-based aggression management program designed to help students increase positive conflict resolution skills, increase the ability to forgive transgressions, and reduce aggressive behavior.

- The *PreVenture Programme: Personality-Targeted Interventions for Adolescent Substance Misuse* is a school-based program designed to prevent alcohol and drug misuse among thirteen- to fifteen-year-old students.

- *Project ALERT* is a school-based prevention program for middle or junior high school students that focuses on alcohol, tobacco, and marijuana use. It seeks to prevent adolescent nonusers from experimenting with these drugs and to prevent youth who are already experimenting from becoming more regular users or abusers.

- *Reconnecting Youth* (RY): *A Peer Group Approach to Building Life Skills* is a school-based prevention program for students from ages fourteen to nineteen that teaches skills to build resiliency against risk factors and control early signs of substance abuse and emotional distress.

- *Responding in Peaceful and Positive Ways* (RiPP) is a school-based violence prevention program for middle school students. It is designed to be implemented along with a peer mediation program. Students practice using a social-cognitive problem-solving model to identify and choose nonviolent strategies for dealing with conflict.

- The *Safe & Civil Schools Positive Behavioral Interventions and Supports* (PBIS) *Model* is a multicomponent, multitiered, comprehensive approach to school-wide improvement. Integrating applied behavior analysis, research on effective schools, and systems change management theory, the intervention is an application of positive behavior support (PBS), a set of strategies or procedures designed to improve behavior by employing positive and systematic techniques.

- The *SANKOFA Youth Violence Prevention Program* is a strengths-based, culturally tailored preventive intervention for African American adolescents from thirteen to nineteen. The goal of this school-based intervention is to equip youth with the knowledge, attitudes, skills, confidence, and motivation to minimize their risk for involvement in violence, victimization owing to violence, and other negative behaviors, such as alcohol and other drug use.

- *Say It Straight* (SIS) is a communication training program designed to help students and adults develop empowering communication skills and behaviors and increase self-awareness, self-efficacy, and personal and social responsibility.

- *Second Step* is a classroom-based social skills program for children from four to fourteen years of age that teaches socioemotional skills aimed at reducing impulsive and aggressive behavior while increasing social competence.

- *SOS Signs of Suicide* is a two-day secondary-school-based intervention that includes screening and education. Students are screened for depression and suicide risk and referred for professional help as indicated.

- *Stay on Track* is a school-based substance abuse prevention curriculum conducted over a three-year period with students in grades six through eight. The intervention is designed to help students assess the risks associated with substance abuse; enhance decision-making, goal-setting, communication, and resistance strategies; improve antidrug normative beliefs and attitudes; and reduce substance use.

- *Storytelling for Empowerment* is a school-based bilingual (English and Spanish) intervention for teenagers at risk for substance abuse, HIV, and other problem behaviors due to living in impoverished communities with high availability of drugs and limited health care services.

- *Students Taking a Right Stand* (STARS) Nashville Student Assistance Program (SAP) is based on an employee assistance model and provides comprehensive school-based prevention services for students in kindergarten through twelfth grade.

- *Teaching Kids to Cope* (TKC) is a cognitive-behavioral health education program, based on stress and coping theory, for adolescents aged twelve to eighteen with depressive symptomatology and/or suicidal ideation. This group treatment program teaches adolescents a range of skills designed to improve their coping with stressful life events and decrease their depressive symptoms.
- *Teenage Health Teaching Modules* (THTM), a school-based health curriculum for students in grades six to twelve, attempts to improve students' immediate and long-term health by influencing their knowledge, attitudes, and behaviors regarding critical adolescent health content areas, including alcohol, tobacco, and other drug use; injury and violence prevention; and mental and emotional health.
- *Too Good for Drugs* (TGFD) is a school-based prevention program for kindergarten through twelfth grade that builds on students' resiliency by teaching them how to be socially competent and autonomous problem solvers.
- *Too Good for Violence* (TGFV) is a school-based violence prevention and character education program for students in kindergarten through twelfth grade. It is designed to enhance pro-social behaviors and skills and improve protective factors related to conflict and violence.
- *Trauma-Focused Coping* (TFC), sometimes called multimodality trauma treatment, is a school-based group intervention for children and adolescents in grades four through twelve who have been exposed to a traumatic stressor (e.g., disaster, violence, murder, suicide, fire, or accident).

Collaborations between school social workers and mental health workers are necessary to effectively intervene in the problems surrounding mental health issues and their impact on education. Working together in a common effort for a common purpose will allow for both effective and efficient uses of resources. Alliances between the school system and the mental health system will move us forward in addressing the prevention and treatment needs of children and families who are at risk of mental health issues. Through creativity, trust, and dedication, school social workers can bring about collaborations that make a difference in the lives of children and families.

REFERENCES

Centers for Disease Control and Prevention. (2014). *Web-based injury statistics query and reporting system (WISQARS)*. Retrieved from http://www.cdc.gov/injury/wisqars /index.html

Individuals with Disabilities Education Act, 20 U.S.C.A. §§ 1400–1485 (2004).

Rehabilitation Act of 1973 (1973). Pub. L. 93–112, 87 Stat. 355 (codified as 29 U.S.C. § 701).

Substance Abuse and Mental Health Services Administration. (2014). *National registry of evidence-based programs and practices*. Available from http://www.nrepp.samhsa .gov/Index.aspx

U.S. Department of Health & Human Services, Children's Bureau. (2008). *School-based child maltreatment programs: Synthesis of lessons learned*. Washington, DC: Author.

Mental Health Resources for Working with Children and Adolescents

ADOLESCENT AND TEEN HEALTH TOPICS

http://www.cdc.gov/HealthyYouth/healthtopics/index.htm

ADOLESCENT DEVELOPMENT

http://fcs.osu.edu/family-life/teens-and-young-adults/parenting-adolescents
http://www.umm.edu/ency/article/002003.htm
https://ufhealth.org/adolescent-development

ADOLESCENT GROWTH AND DEVELOPMENT

http://www.ext.vt.edu/topics/family/child-development/index.html

ADOLESCENT HEALTH AND DEVELOPMENT

http://www.who.int/maternal_child_adolescent/topics/adolescence/second
-decade/en/

BRAIN

http://www.nimh.nih.gov/health/educational-resources/brain-basics/brain
-basics.shtml

CHILD AND ADOLESCENT DEVELOPMENT

http://www.themediaproject.com/facts/development/index.htm

CHILD AND TEEN HEALTH

http://www.nlm.nih.gov/medlineplus/childandteenhealth.html

GIRL POWER—NATIONAL PUBLIC EDUCATION CAMPAIGN

https://www.ncjrs.gov/App/publications/abstract.aspx?ID=172442

GIRLS' HEALTH

http://girlshealth.gov

MENTAL HEALTH

http://www.samhsa.gov/treatment

NATIONAL ADOLESCENT HEALTH INFORMATION CENTER

http://nahic.ucsf.edu/

NORMAL ADOLESCENT DEVELOPMENT

http://life.familyeducation.com/puberty/growth-and-development/36357.html
http://www.aacap.org/AACAP/Families_and_Youth/Facts_for_Families/Home.aspx

POSITIVE YOUTH DEVELOPMENT

http://www.acf.hhs.gov/sites/default/files/fysb/whatispyd20120829.pdf

STAGES OF ADOLESCENT DEVELOPMENT

http://www.childdevelopmentinfo.com/development/teens_stages.shtml

TEEN DEVELOPMENT

http://www.nlm.nih.gov/medlineplus/teendevelopment.html
http://kidshealth.org/teen

TEEN HEALTH CENTER

http://teenshealth.org/teen

TEEN MENTAL HEALTH

http://www.nlm.nih.gov/medlineplus/teenmentalhealth.html

TEENS' PAGE

http://www.nlm.nih.gov/medlineplus/teenspage.html

TEENAGE HEALTH

http://healthfinder.gov/HealthTopics/Population/pre-teens-and-teens

YOUTH DEVELOPMENT LINKS

http://ncfy.acf.hhs.gov

Index

Note: Page numbers followed by "t" refer to tables.

About the Authors

Kirstin Painter, PhD, LCSW, is senior director of research for Mental Health Mental Retardation of Tarrant County, a community mental health and substance abuse center, and research associate at the Center for Child Welfare, School of Social Work, University of Texas at Arlington. She is lead evaluator on several state and federally funded research projects. She oversees a team of evaluators whose specialty is conducting longitudinal studies of vulnerable populations relating to homelessness, HIV, substance abuse, and chronic mental illness. She also has extensive administrative and clinical expertise in community mental health working with youth and their families.

Maria Scannapieco, PhD, MSW, is professor at the School of Social Work, University of Texas at Arlington, and director of the Center for Child Welfare. She has worked in the public child welfare arena for thirty years as an educator and researcher, with direct child protection and foster care administrative experience. Since 1996, she has received more than $1 million a year in state and federal grants for training programs, curriculum development, technical assistance, and research. She has extensive experience in grant development, implementation, management, and dissemination. She is the editor of *Kinship Foster Care: Policy, Practice, and Research* (1999), with Rebecca L. Hegar, and author of *Understanding Child Maltreatment: An Ecological and Developmental Perspective* (2005), with Kelli Connell-Carrick, and many articles on the impact of child maltreatment on mental health, out-of-home placement, preparation for adult living programs, and training and retention of child welfare workers.